The Profession of Dietetics

A Team Approach

June Payne-Palacio
Pepperdine University

Deborah D. Canter
Kansas State University

Merrill,
an imprint of Prentice Hall
Englewood Cliffs, New Jersey   *Columbus, Ohio*

Library of Congress Cataloging-in-Publication Data

Payne-Palacio, June

The profession of dietetics : a team approach / June Payne-Palacio,
Deborah D. Canter.

p. cm.

Includes bibliographical references and index.

ISBN 0-02-392394-6

1. Dietetics.   I. Canter, Deborah D.   II. Title.

RM218.5.P39   1996

613.2—dc20   95-25232
                                                  CIP

Editor: Kevin M. Davis
Production Editor: Stephen C. Robb
Design Coordinator: Julia Zonneveld Van Hook
Text Designer: Anne D. Flanagan
Cover Designer: Anne D. Flanagan
Production Manager: Pamela D. Bennett
Electronic Text Management: Marilyn Wilson Phelps, Matthew Williams,
    Karen L. Bretz, Tracey Ward
Illustrations: Karen Bretz

This book was set in Bookman and Swiss by Prentice Hall and was printed
and bound by Quebecor Printing/Book Press. The cover was printed by
Phoenix Color Corp.

 © 1996 by Prentice-Hall, Inc.
A Simon & Schuster Company
Englewood Cliffs, New Jersey 07632

Printed in the United States of America

10 9 8 7 6 5 4 3 2 1

ISBN: 0-02-392394-6

Prentice-Hall International (UK) Limited, *London*
Prentice-Hall of Australia Pty. Limited, *Sydney*
Prentice-Hall Canada, Inc., *Toronto*
Prentice-Hall Hispanoamericana, S. A., *Mexico*
Prentice-Hall of India Private Limited, *New Delhi*
Prentice-Hall of Japan, Inc., *Tokyo*
Simon & Schuster Asia Pte. Ltd., *Singapore*
Editora Prentice-Hall do Brasil, Ltda., *Rio de Janeiro*

Preface

This book is written for students interested in finding out more about the profession of dietetics. Understanding who dietitians are, what dietitians do, and how one becomes a dietitian is a complex task. Few other professions offer so many educational routes for entry or so many ways to practice one's trade. While this diversity is a strength, it often confuses those who wish to enter the profession, as well as prospective customers who are trying to understand who dietitians are and why they should consult one.

It is the goal of this book to present a clear and up-to-date picture of the dietetics profession and try to answer some basic questions:

- What is a profession and how does dietetics qualify as a profession?
- How has the history of the profession shaped dietetics practice today?
- Who are members of the dietetics team and how do they work together?
- What is the American Dietetic Association and why should one be a member?
- What is credentialing of dietetics professionals and why is it important?
- What kinds of positions are filled by dietitians?

- What does the future hold for dietetics practice?

The profession of dietetics is dynamic, exciting, and in need of enthusiastic, energetic, and visionary men and women who wish to join the team. It is our hope that this book enlightens, informs, and inspires those who read it. If this happens, then our dream for this book will have been achieved.

ACKNOWLEDGMENTS

The authors thank the following reviewers for their insightful suggestions: Rebecca L. Bradley, University of Alabama, Birmingham; Dorothy Pond-Smith, Washington State University; Martha L. Taylor, University of North Carolina, Greensboro.

Contents

Chapter 3   The American Dietetic Association   67

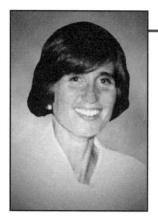

Joyce Gilbert

Gilbert Associates
Nutrition Consultants
Gainesville, Florida

M y name is Joyce Gilbert, and I own a nutrition consulting business in Gainesville, Florida. I attended the University of South Carolina on a basketball scholarship and earned a bachelor's degree in biology and biochemistry. I first learned about dietetics while working on a master's degree in Human Nutrition at Clemson University. It was there that I began to see the applicability of biochemistry to human health. The introduction to the field of nutrition and the profession of dietetics blended two philosophies in my life: to treat learning as a continuum, and to share knowledge.

After earning my master's degree, I completed a supervised practice experience at the South Carolina Department of Mental Health. My career as a research dietitian began at a teaching/research psychiatric facility. Later, my position expanded to include clinical nutrition, and I began a consulting business in sports nutrition. My first contract was the University of South Carolina Women's Athletics Department. I then moved into a management position as director of food and nutritional services, combining clinical dietetics with food systems management. During all this, I maintained my consulting business.

Since my goal was to obtain a Ph.D., I accepted the chance to become a clinical instructor at the University of Florida while working on a doctorate. After completing my doctoral degree, I joined the nutrition faculty of Pennsylvania State University in hopes of continuing my research, teaching, and program development. Family commitments brought me back to Florida, where I have my own consulting business in Gainesville.

The best thing about my current position is the variety. Consulting introduces me to many places and experiences. I've worked at the National Aeronautics and Space Administration (NASA) on research aimed at establishing the micronutrient needs of humans in microgravity conditions. I've worked with the U.S. military on research protocols to evaluate the effects of environment on micronutrient status. I work with elite athletes at the university and Olympic level, have a disordered eating clinic, and work with AIDS patients. I also consult in pediatric diabetes, in drug/alcohol rehabilitation, and with mentally challenged individuals.

Dietetics parallels my life philosophy: to touch many lives with my given talents, by being a positive influence and by making a difference. I believe in living life proactively. The challenge of blending science and health—and using this knowledge to help prevent disease—is an attractive aspect of dietetics. Though dietetics may be very broad in its scope, it does not lose sight of the individual. True education both imparts knowledge and gives individuals the tools necessary to continue learning and developing skills. Dietetics does this.

Focus, discover, learn, share, and remember to give something back to humankind. Do what you love, for you will always do that best.

CHAPTER 1

The Profession of Dietetics

WHAT IS DIETETICS?

This is an exciting time to be a nutrition professional. The knowledge that life-style choices, such as diet and exercise, can make a dramatic difference in quality of life is becoming more widespread. People are eager for information that can give them an edge in competitive sports, improve physical appearance, make them feel better, and help them live longer, more productive lives. The knowledge that what we eat can dramatically affect our health will create a demand for those who can provide this information. It is predicted that by the year 2000, seven of the ten fastest-growing occupations will be in health-related fields.[1] Dietetics is predicted to be among the twenty fastest-growing careers, with a projected growth rate of 28 percent and an average salary of $70,000.[2] Sports nutrition, in particular, has been singled out as one of the twenty-five hottest careers.[3]

Perhaps no other profession offers such diversity of opportunity as the field of dietetics does today. Early dietetic practitioners were usually found in an institutional kitchen. Today, as Figure 1.1 attests, dietitians can be found almost anywhere. Dietetic practitioners may work in private practice or in a hospital, with patients referred by physicians for help in implementing necessary nutritional modifications. Dietetic practitioners serve as consultants in corporate wellness programs, weight-loss programs, and eating disorder clinics. Professional athletes and athletic teams often have full-time dietitians on their training staffs.

Dietetic practitioners are also involved in scientific research and education. Increasing numbers of dietitians have careers in sales, marketing, and public relations for the food industry, pharmaceutical and computer companies, and equipment manufacturers. They are involved in many areas of community work, especially with pregnant women, women with infants and young children, and the elderly.

Dietetic practitioners are particularly qualified to manage foodservice operations in hospitals, nursing homes, colleges and universities, public schools, com-

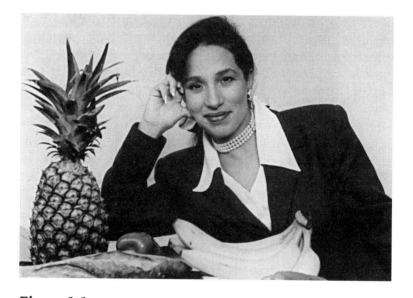

Figure 1.1
Evelyn Tribole, M.S., R.D., has her own private practice, is the author of several books, teaches, serves as an ambassador for The American Dietetic Association, is a sports nutrition consultant, and appears regularly on "Good Morning, America."
Source: Courtesy of Craig Sjodin/ABC Photography Department.

mercial restaurants, correctional facilities, catering operations, airline commissaries, and community programs (Figure 1.2).

Although dietetic practitioners are regarded as experts in nutrition, there is still a lack of recognition from the public. And while the American public has increased its knowledge and understanding of foods and nutrition, misinformation still abounds. Popular magazines are full of attention-grabbing, but inaccurate, advice. Health-food stores promote the sale of supposed "super nutrients," to the tune of billions of dollars a year. The general public lacks the educational background to discern a good study from a poor one. Many people still don't know that you can't believe everything you read. Some common warning signs of nutritional quackery are listed and described in Figure 1.3.

The basis of dietetics is the firm belief that optimal nutrition is essential for the health and well-being of every person. This is why dietetics is an integral com-

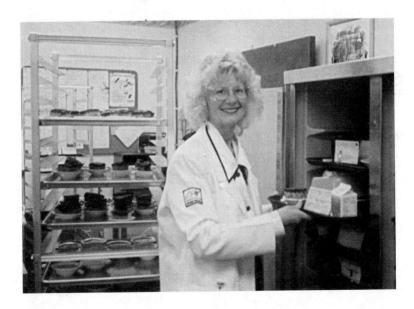

Figure 1.2
A dietary manager checks patient trays for accuracy.
Source: Photo courtesy of Doris Douglas, CDM.

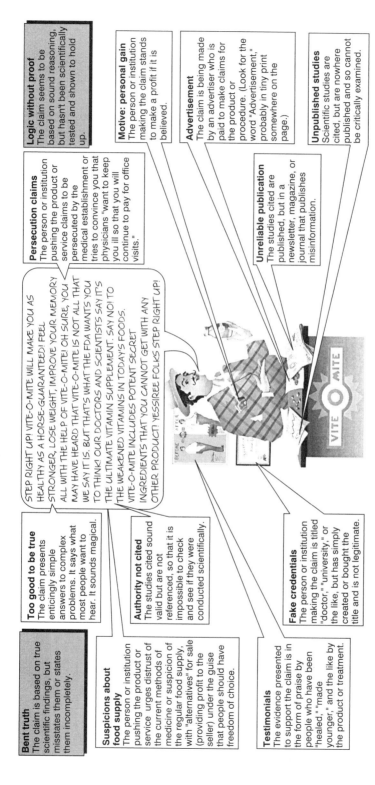

Figure 1.3

The warning signs of nutritional quackery.

Source: Reprinted by permission from page 25 of *Nutrition Concepts and Controversies* by Frances Sizer and Eleanor Whitney; Copyright © 1994 by West Publishing Company. All rights reserved.

ponent of the health-care field. Nutritional support helps return patients to health and keep them that way. A team effort by doctors, nurses, and dietitians is usually necessary to return a patient to health.

The words *food* and *nutrition* are not synonymous. Food is the main source of nourishment, which is influenced by a complex array of internal and external factors. When food cannot be used to achieve nutrition, intravenous feeding or total parenteral nutrition (TPN) become important.

Societal needs are best served by having a population that is adequately nourished. Dietetics serves people by offering correct and current information so that individuals can make their own choices. The education, training, and knowledge of dietitians make them uniquely qualified to help individuals and society to meet nutritional needs.

WHAT IS A PROFESSION?

What is a profession, and how does dietetics qualify as a profession? One generic definition might be "A profession is an occupation for which preliminary training is intellectual in character, involving knowledge and learning as distinguished from mere skill, which is pursued largely for others and not merely for one's self, and in which financial return is not an accepted measure of success." The goals committee of The American Dietetic Association interprets a profession as a calling requiring:

- specialized knowledge and often long and intensive preparation;
- instruction in skills and methods as well as scientific, historical, or scholarly principles underlying such skills and methods;
- maintenance, by force of organization or concerted opinion, of high standards of achievement and conduct;

- commitment of its members to continued study; and
- a kind of work which has as its primary purpose the rendering of a public service.

A professional is one who represents or belongs to a profession.[4]

HOW IS DIETETICS A PROFESSION?

Five main characteristics of dietetic practice qualify it for professional status:

1. a specialized body of knowledge;
2. specialized services rendered to society;
3. an obligation for service to the client which overrides personal considerations;
4. concern for competence and honor among the practitioners, and
5. an obligation for continuing education, research, and sharing of knowledge for the common good.

A dietitian has been defined as "a professional person who is a translator of the science and art of foods, nutrition, and dietetics in the service of people—whether individually or in families or larger groups; healthy or sick; and at all stages of the life cycle."[5] Dietetic practice is defined as the application of principles derived from the integration of knowledge of food, nutrition, biochemistry, physiology, management, and behavioral and social science to achieve and maintain the health of people.[6] See Figure 1.4 for a graphic depiction of the different fields integrated by dietitians.

A BRIEF HISTORY OF DIETETICS

Ancient History

Dietetics has not always enjoyed professional status, but the role of food in curing, preventing, or causing

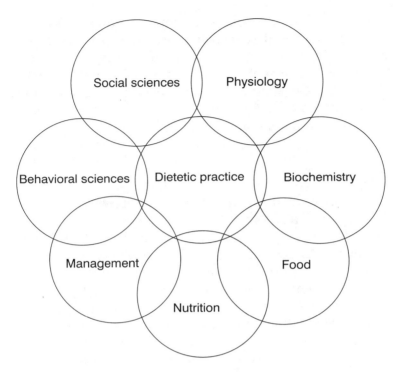

Figure 1.4
Dietetic practice.

illness has been recognized since the beginning of recorded history. "If a man has pain inside, food and drink coming back to his mouth . . . let him refrain from eating onions for three days" is the first known written dietary recommendation, carved on Babylonian stone tablets about 2500 B.C.[7] The typical daily regimen during this time consisted of barley paste or bread, onions, a few beans, and beer. The Book of Judges in the Old Testament contains a prenatal dietary prescription that has withstood the test of time: "Therefore beware, and drink no wine or strong drink, and eat nothing unclean, for lo, you shall conceive and bear a son."[8]

The word *diet* is from the Greek *diaita* meaning "manner of living."[9] It appears in many early writings, including those of Hippocrates and Galen.[10] The oldest known cookbook, *Apicius*, (approximately 100 B.C.) contains many dietetic principles that are still sound today.[11] In ancient China, food therapy was practiced as a special branch of medicine.[12] Chinese observations about diabetes date to the third century,[13] and descriptions of night blindness and its correct dietary cure date to the seventh century.[14]

The Middle Ages

Hospital records from St. Bartholomew's Hospital, founded in Britain in 1123, provide the first written evidence of a typical hospital menu. Bread and beer formed the basis of the diet.[15] This obviously inadequate and unpalatable diet led to a prevalence of scurvy among patients. Other conditions in early British hospitals were also poor. Sanitation was nonexistent, there was overcrowding, buildings were unsafe, and stern disciplinary measures were used on noncompliant patients.

With the publication of *De re Medicina* in 1478 in Florence, diet became an important part of medical practice. In this publication, medicine was divided into three branches—diseases treated manually, diseases treated by medicine, and diseases treated by diet. In 1480, the first printed cookbook appeared, containing reference to quality and varieties of meat, fish, fruits, and vegetables, how they nourish the body, and how they should be prepared.[16]

Progress in the Eighteenth and Nineteenth Centuries

Until the eighteenth century, beliefs and writings about diet were based on insufficient scientific evidence. But with advances in chemistry and physics came the foundation necessary to establish dietetics as a profession. Lavoisier's work on digestion is generally regarded as the first modern, scientific experiments on nutrition.[17]

Still, progress was slow. A patient in an English hospital in the eighteenth century would receive the only menu served:

Four to five ounces of meat (usually already boiled for the broth)

Three-quarters to one pound of bread

Two to three pints of beer

Pottage or pudding

Fruits and vegetables were missing from this daily allowance—they were suspected by some as being harmful and by others as having medicinal, rather than nutritive value. Small amounts of cheese, butter, roots, and greens were sometimes included in the daily fare. Family and friends could bring food to supplement the meager hospital offerings, or patients could buy food from the food sellers who came through the wards.

The most expensive item on the menu was the beer. Doctors of the time believed that alcohol was necessary to treat illness. Since water was contaminated, beer was used extensively. When cost-cutting measures were instituted, the beer allowance was reduced or completely eliminated.

Patients who were unable to eat the full diet or complained about the food were disciplined. Punishments included cutting the food allowance in half, omitting some meals entirely, or restricting patients to toast and water for a week.[18]

In American hospitals too, food was given little thought and conditions were very poor. The first hospitals in the United States were in Philadelphia—Philadelphia General Hospital was built in 1731, and Pennsylvania Hospital was built in 1751.[19] Mush and molasses was the usual fare, with a pint of beer included for supper.[20] After the War of 1812, fruit was added to the menu as a garnish.

There was little improvement in hospital conditions until the humanitarian movement of the late nineteenth century. Great progress was made between 1850 and 1920.

Florence Nightingale (1820–1910), a superintendent of nurses in English military hospitals in Turkey during the Crimean War (1854–1856), established foodservice for the troops (Figure 1.5). With the help of a French chef, Alexis Soyer, she reduced the death rate of injured soldiers by improving diet and sanitary conditions. Later, in her writings and nursing practice, Nightingale continued to demonstrate her belief in the importance of nutrition and foodservice management by emphasizing the selection and service of food and the art and science of feeding the sick.[21]

Sarah Tyson Rorer (1849–1937) is considered to be the first American dietitian (Figure 1.6). Her training consisted of some medical school lectures and a three-month cooking course. In 1878 Sarah Rorer opened the Philadelphia Cooking School, where students learned about food values, protein, and carbohydrates, but nothing about calories and vitamins. Students took ten classes in chemistry, several on physiology and hygiene, and ten classes on cooking for the sick.

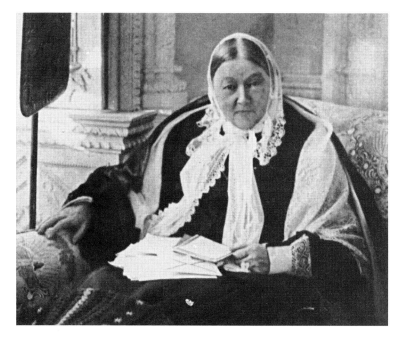

Figure 1.5
Florence Nightingale.
Source: Courtesy of the Florence Nightingale Museum, London.

Twelve students graduated each year for 33 years, and they secured positions planning meals and supervising production in hospital kitchens.[22]

In 1877, the American Medical Association formed a Committee on Dietetics, and asked Rorer to edit a new publication entitled *The Dietetic Gazette*.[23] Later, she published *Household News* on her own, in which she wrote articles on topics such as feeding the sick and designing a kitchen and answered questions regarding diet from readers.[24] In her lifetime, she wrote more than fifty books and booklets, and wrote articles for such magazines as *Ladies' Home Journal*, *Table Talk*, and *Good Housekeeping*.[25] Rorer also established the

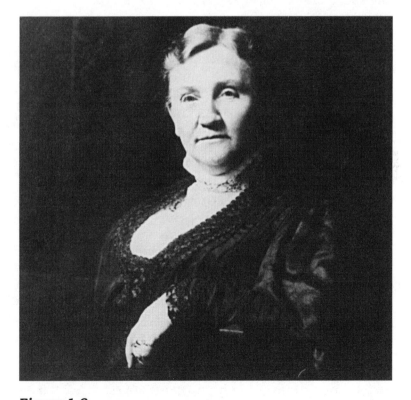

Figure 1.6
Sarah Tyson Rorer.
Source: Photo courtesy of The American Dietetic Association.

first diet kitchen and dietary counseling service, at the request of three well-known physicians.

In 1896, the United States Department of Agriculture published *Bulletin 28*, the first food composition tables.[26] It was an indispensable resource for dietetic practitioners for many years.

At the Lake Placid Conference on Home Economics in 1899, the term *dietitian* was first defined. The conference attendees determined that the title *dietitian* should be "applied to persons who specialize in the knowledge of food and can meet the demands of the medical profession for diet therapy."[27]

The Young Profession in the Twentieth Century

The Iowa Agricultural School in Ames was probably the first college to offer courses in cookery, in 1872. A yearly course in "household chemistry," which included cookery, was begun in 1877 at the Kansas State Agricultural College in Manhattan.[28] Other colleges and universities soon followed their lead. The first internship for dietitians was established by Florence Corbett in 1903, at the New York Department of Charities. Applicants for the three-month course had to be over 25 years of age, have taught for one year, and be domestic science graduates.

At about the same time, Casimir Funk discovered a chemical substance named *amine*. Since this substance appeared essential to life, he added the prefix *vita*.[29] Discovery of the individual vitamines would come much later, but this initial discovery was a milepost in nutritional history.

In 1910, dietitians were practicing in poorly defined roles with a diversity of titles, but they were facing some of the same problems that dietitians face today. Few people could define the role of the dietist, dietician, dietitian, or nutrition worker, as dietitians were variously called. The title *nutritionist* appeared in the early 1920s, and the spelling *dietitian* was agreed upon in 1930.[30]

Fighting faddism and quackery was an issue in 1910, just as it is today. Fletcherizing, or chewing each mouthful of food 32 times before swallowing, is an example of a harmless but ineffective popular notion of that day. Calorie counting, high protein or low protein diets, and natural foods were other popular fads.

Nutritional research received an unexpected boost in importance with the outbreak of World War I. The examination of 2.5 million military draftees in Great Britain in 1917 found 41 percent to be in poor health and unfit for military duty, due most commonly to nutritional status.[31] In the United States, the American Red Cross enrolled dietitians for army duty. Three hundred and fifty-six dietitians served in World War I. Mary de Garmo Bryan, who later became the second president of The American Dietetic Association, was among them (Figures 1.7, 1.8, 1.9, and 1.10). The nutritional expertise of these brave dietitians provided leadership for both the nourishment of hospitalized soldiers and the general public at home. Conservation of food was encouraged, as dietitians advised the government on efficient methods of food production, distribution, and preparation (Figure 1.11).

When the American Home Economic Association decided not to hold its annual meeting in 1917 because of the war, two dietitians, Lenna Frances Cooper (Figure 1.12) and Lulu G. Graves, organized a special meeting of hospital dietitians to discuss emergency war needs. Out of this meeting of 98 people The American Dietetic Association (ADA) was formed. This association, with 39 charter members and dues of $1 per year, was formed to address the interests of dietitians. Its first president was Lulu Graves (Figure 1.13) who was head of the dietary department at Lakeside Hospital in Cleveland (Figure 1.14). The first meeting of ADA was held in the basement at Lakeside Hospital. Graves served as president for the first three years. Lenna Frances Cooper served as first vice president. The continuing history of ADA will be covered in Chapter 3 and the history of education of dietetic practitioners, in Chapter 5.

Dieto-therapy as practiced in the early 1900s consisted of many special diets like the Sippy Diet for ulcers, which consisted of cream and poached eggs. Diabetic diets varied widely even after the discovery of insulin in 1921.

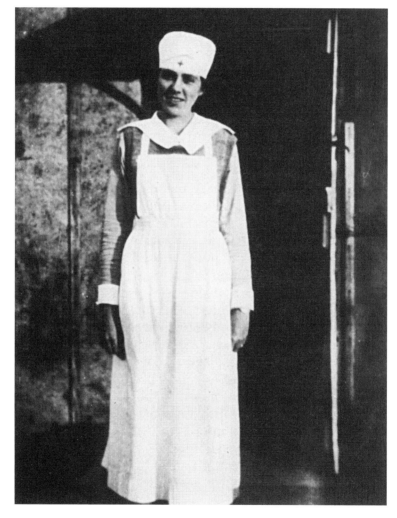

Figure 1.7
Mary de Garmo Bryan in 1917, wearing an American Red Cross uniform in France.
Source: Photo courtesy of The American Dietetic Association.

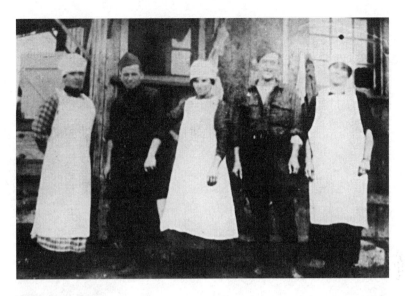

Figure 1.8
Mary de Garmo Bryan and a field kitchen staff during World War I.
Source: Photo courtesy of The American Dietetic Association.

The passage of the federal Maternity and Infancy Act in the 1920s allowed state health departments to employ nutritionists.[32] The passage of Title V of the Social Security Act in 1935 provided major impetus for the employment of nutrition consultants in state and local health departments by making federal funds available for this purpose.[33]

The profession of dietetics continued to become more widely recognized and broaden in scope. World War II contributed to the public recognition of the role of dietitians: nearly 2,000 dietitians were commissioned in the armed services, while many others educated the public at home (Figures 1.15, 1.16, and 1.17). The practice of dietetics broadened to include institutions such as restaurants, airlines, and industrial plants. After the war, dietitians were granted full military status and their position in the healthcare setting strengthened with the emphasis on allied health professions and the healthcare team concept.[34]

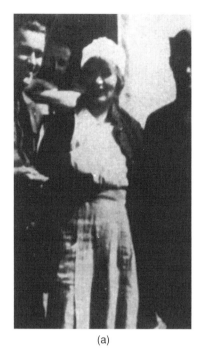 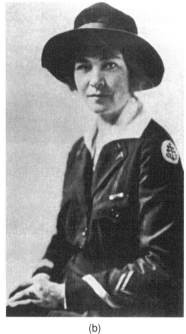

(a)   (b)

Figure 1.9
Dietitians' Red Cross uniforms from World War I: (a) a duty uniform of blue crepe with Red Cross cape and (b) a gray travel uniform.
Source: Photos courtesy of The American Dietetic Association.

Passage of the National School Lunch Act in 1946 expanded dietetics to include the establishment of school lunch programs, including the training of personnel in foodservice and nutrition education. The Hill–Burton Hospital Facilities Survey and Construction Act (1946) and the Medicare and Medicaid legislation of the 1960s created demand for the services of consultant dietitians in healthcare facilities such as nursing homes. The civil rights movement of the 1960s brought the issues of poverty and hunger into the political spotlight. The government instituted its war on poverty, and Senator Hubert Humphrey worked with the Senate Select Committee on Nutrition and Human Needs.[35] As a result of these and other efforts, the

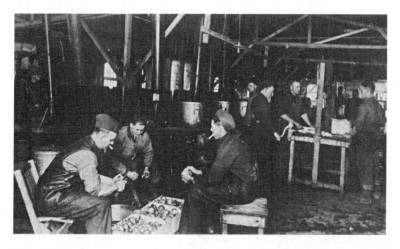

Figure 1.10
General kitchen and mess hall, Savenay, France, 1919.
Source: Photo courtesy of The American Dietetic Association.

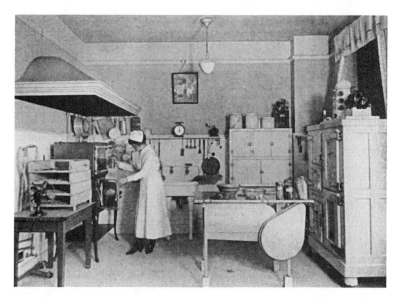

Figure 1.11
Mary E. Pascoe, dietitian for the New York Edison Company
(now Consolidated Edison), demonstrating the correct
method for drying food in an electric oven in 1917. Note
utensils of the period and one of the first domestic
refrigerators.
Source: Courtesy of the Consolidated Edison Co. of New York, Inc.

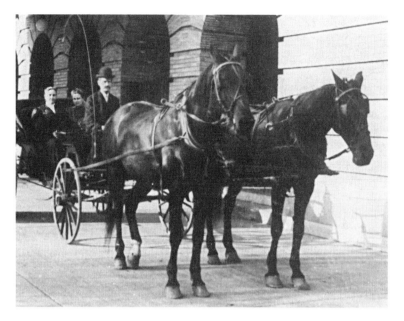

Figure 1.12
Lenna Frances Cooper (in carriage, right) and Sarah Tyson
Rorer (in carriage, middle) in 1916.
Source: Photo courtesy of The American Dietetic Association.

United States Department of Agriculture's (USDA) food
assistance programs to low-income families were
established or expanded in the 1970s. Important
among these were the food stamp program and school
lunch and breakfast programs; child care and summer
foodservice for children; supplemental feeding programs for women, infants, and children (WIC); and
nutrition for the elderly.[36]
Food assistance programs have developed more
rapidly and with more support than nutrition education programs. In 1968, the Cooperative Extension
Service of the USDA began the Expanded Food and
Nutrition Education Program (EFNEP), which provides
nutrition and food education for low-income families.
In 1975, three years after the start of the WIC program,
an education component was legislated. And, in 1977,
nutrition education was incorporated into the food
stamp program. The Food And Agriculture Act of 1977

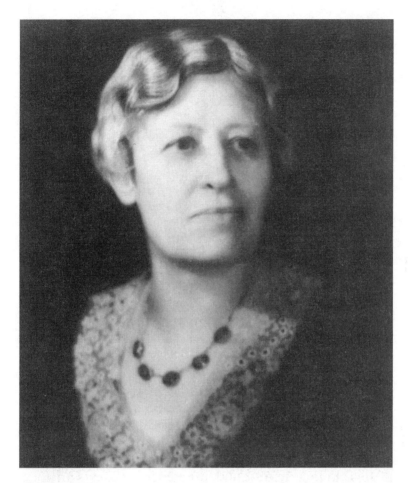

Figure 1.13
Lulu Graves
Source: Photo courtesy of The American Dietetic Association.

included the Nutrition Education and Training Program (NETP), the first federal nutrition program for children.[37] The ADA and others express the need for making nutrition education a primary component of *all* food assistance programs.[38]

Facing the Twenty-First Century

Today, dietetics is an honored profession with members striving to achieve the highest professional stan-

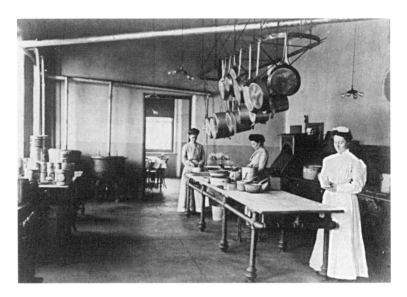

Figure 1.14
Lakeside Hospital kitchen, 1905. The first meeting of The
American Dietetic Association was held here in 1917.
Source: Photo courtesy of University Hospitals, Cleveland.

dards of integrity, service, competence, and vision. Two
leaders of the profession wrote recently: "Our profession today is marked by achievement and change. . . .
[We] have come a long way in a relatively short period
of time. We have become valued professional members
of health-care teams and recognized experts in food
and nutrition, food service management, and wellness. . . . We need the courage to perceive ourselves
succeeding in new roles, to attract a diversity of people
to dietetics, and to polish and practice marketing,
management, leadership, and sales skills."[39]

Change is rapid in all areas of the dietetics profession—education, research, and practice. The leading
issue facing the profession at the present time is
healthcare reform. Debate continues over the funda-
mental changes proposed for the way the nation reim-
burses health-care services. Health-care reform presents both an opportunity and a challenge to the
profession.

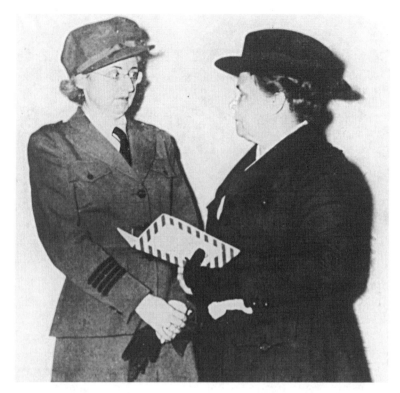

Figure 1.15
Lenna Frances Cooper (left) in a World War I uniform and
Helen Burns (right) in a World War II uniform at the twenty-
fifth anniversary of The American Dietetic Association in
1942.
Source: Photo courtesy of The American Dietetic Association.

Increased emphasis is being placed on nutrition and
women's health with the recognition of the link
between nutrition and the three major diseases that
affect women—heart disease, breast cancer, and osteoporosis. The inadequacy of nutrition education in medical schools is another concern—eight of the ten leading diseases in the United States are linked to
nutrition. The gap between consumer nutrition knowledge and behavior presents another opportunity for
dietetic practitioners. In the commercial/retail foodservice market, dietetic professionals are an underuti-

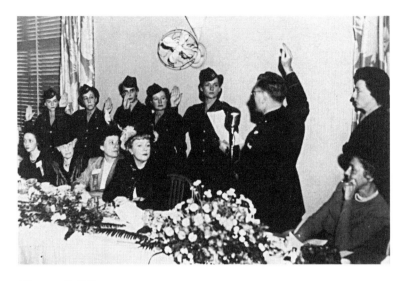

Figure 1.16
Army dietitians receive permanent rank, 1947.
Source: Photo courtesy of The American Dietetic Association.

lized resource: it is predicted that, by the year 2000, Americans will spend 50 cents of every food dollar eating away from home.[40] The development of leadership among the members of the profession is another current priority. A number of dynamic and dedicated individuals have emerged to assume leadership roles, and will continue to do so as the profession matures.[41]

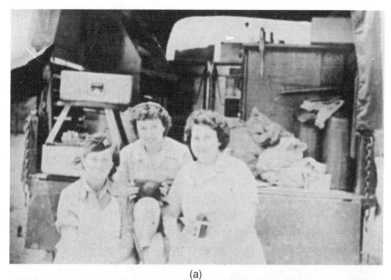

(a)

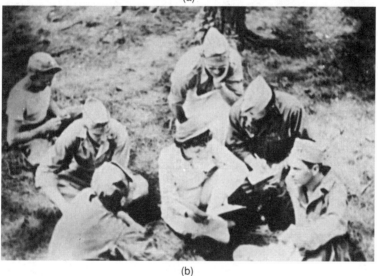

(b)

Figure 1.17
Equipment changes in a field kitchen in World War II, but
dietitians teach anytime and anywhere.
Source: Photos courtesy of The American Dietetic Association.

SUMMARY

"The world is happier, healthier, [and] better off because of the work you do," proclaimed Rabbi Harold S. Kushner to the dietetic professionals gathered at the 1991 ADA Annual Meeting.[42] The work of dietetics is considered a profession because it requires a specialized body of knowledge; members render specialized services to society; their obligations to serve override personal considerations; and competence, honor, continuing education, research, and sharing of knowledge for the common good are considered necessary.

Dietetic practice combines the disciplines of food, nutrition, biochemistry, physiology, management, and the behavioral and social sciences to achieve and maintain health. The dietetic professional applies the science and art of foods, nutrition, and dietetics to the service of people.

Although there is a long history of the relationship of food to health, the profession is very young. Much of the progress has been made in the last one hundred years. Advances in scientific research, legislation, social and economic factors, military conflicts, and the leadership of some dynamic and dedicated dietitians contributed to the advancement of the profession.

In closing his remarks, Rabbi Kushner said, "You each have the power to change the world. Not in a super-dramatic way, not with headlines and Nobel Prizes, but with deeds of caring that affect and improve other people's lives. . . . This is what you are doing every day at work and [you are] changing the world thereby."[43]

SUGGESTED ACTIVITIES

1. Read one of the autobiographies in *Legends and Legacies* (C. E. Vickery and N. Cotugna, Kendall/Hunt Publishing, 1990) and give an oral report to your class.

2. Secure a very old book on health or cooking from a library or used bookstore. Compare its content to present-day beliefs and practices.

3. Interview a fifty-year member of the profession to obtain a personal history of changes that have occurred.

4. Read a journal article chronicling the history of dietetic practice during World War I or II. For example:

   Hodges PAM. Perspective on history: Military dietetics in Europe during World War I. *Journal of American Dietetics Association*, 1993;93:897–900.

   or

   Hodges PAM. Perspectives on history: Military dietetics in the Philippines during World War II. *Journal of American Dietetics Association*, 1992;92:840–843.

NOTES

1. Snelling RO, Snelling, AM. *Jobs*! New York: Fireside/Simon & Schuster; 1992.

2. Brown N. Careers 2000: Where will the jobs be? *Los Angeles Times*, May 5, 1991.

3. Russell AM. Twenty-five hottest careers. *Working Woman*, 1989; 67.

4. The American Dietetic Association Committee on Goals of Education for Dietetics, Goals of the lifetime education of the dietitian. *Journal of the American Dietetic Association*, 1969;54:91–93.

5. Galbraith A. Excellence defined. *Journal of the American Dietetic Association*, 1975;67:211.

6. South ML. Charting for the changing scene. In Vaden, AG, ed. *Charting for the Changing Scene*. Chicago: American Dietetic Association; 1981.

7. Jastrow M. *The Civilization of Babylonia and Assyria*. Philadelphia: J.B. Lippincott Company, 1915.

8. *The Bible* (revised standard version). New York: Collins, 1971.

9. Gove PB, ed. *Webster's Third New International Dictionary*. Springfield, MA: G & C Merriam Co., 1971.

10. Barber MI, ed. *History of the American Dietetic Association* (1917–1959). Philadelphia: J.B. Lippincott Co., 1959.

11. Vehling JD, trans. *Apicius: Cooking and Dining in Imperial Rome*. Chicago: Walter M. Hill, 1936.

12. Whang J. Chinese traditional food therapy. *Journal of the American Dietetic Association*, 1981;78:55–57.

13. Durant W. *Our Oriental Heritage*. New York: Simon and Schuster, 1935.

14. Garrison FH. *An Introduction to the History of Medicine*. 4th ed. Philadelphia: W.B. Saunders Co., 1967.

15. Isch C. A history of hospital fare. In: Beeuwkes AM, Todhunter EN, Weigley ES, eds. Essays on the History of Nutrition and Dietetics. Chicago: American Dietetic Association, 1967.

16. De Honesta Voluptate. (In Whitcomb M, ed. *Literary Source Book of the Italian Renaissance*. Philadelphia, 1900.)

17. Needham J. Clerks and craftsmen in China and the West. In: *Lectures and Addresses on the History of Science and Technology*. Cambridge, MA: Cambridge University Press, 1970.

18. Rabenn WB. Hospital diets in eighteenth century England. In: Beeuwkes AM, Todhunter EN, Weigley ES, eds. *Essays on the History of Nutrition and Dietetics*. Chicago: American Dietetic Association, 1967.

19. See Note 15, above.

20. The American Dietetic Association Study Commission on Dietetics. *A New Look at the Profession of Dietetics*. Chicago: American Dietetic Association, 1984.

21. Cooper LF. Florence Nightingale's contribution to dietetics. In: Beeuwkes AM, Todhunter EN, Weigley ES, eds. *Essays on the History of Nutrition and Dietetics*. Chicago: American Dietetic Association, 1967.

22. Cooper LF. The dietitian and her profession. *Journal of the American Dietetic Association*, 1938;14:751–758.

23. Rorer ST. Early dietetics. *Journal of the American Dietetics Association*, 1934;x:289.

24. Rorer ST. Feeding the sick. *Household News*, 1893;1:69. Rorer ST. How to design a kitchen. *Household News*, 1894;2:17. Rorer ST. Answers to inquiries. *Household News*, 1893;1:13.

25. Weigley ES. Sarah Tyson Rorer: First American dietitian? *Journal of the American Dietetic Association*, 1980;77:11–15.

26. Atwater WO, Bryant AP. *The Chemical Composition of American Food Materials*. U.S. Department of Agriculture Bulletin No. 28. Washington, D.C.: U.S. Government Printing Office, 1896.

27. Corbett FR. The training of dietitians for hospitals. *Journal of Home Economics*, 1909;1:62.

28. Gilson HE. Some historical notes on the development of diet therapy. In Beeuwkes AM, Todhunter EN, Weigley ES, eds. *Essays on the History of Nutrition and Dietetics*. Chicago: American Dietetic Association, 1967.

29. Funk C. The etiology of the deficiency diseases. *Journal of State Medicine*, 1912;341–368.

30. Egan MC. Public health nutrition services: Issues today and tomorrow. *Journal of the American Dietetic Association*, 1980;77:423.

31. Burnett J. *Plenty and Want: A Social History of Diet in England from 1815 to the Present Day*. London: Nelson, 1966.

32. See Note 30, above.

33. See Note 30, above. Also, Eliot MM, Heseltine, MM. Nutrition in maternal and child health programs. *Nutrition Review*, 1947;533–35.

34. See Note 10, above.

35. Bray GA. Nutrition in the Humphrey tradition. *Journal of the American Dietetic Association*, 1979;75:116–121.

36. Cross AT. USDA's strategies for the 80s: Nutrition education. *Journal of the American Dietetic Association*, 1980;76:333–337.

37. See Note 36, above.

38. ADA testifies in favor of improving USDA domestic feeding programs. *ADA Courier*, 1993;32:2.

39. Calvert-Finn S, Rinke, W. Probing the envelope of Dietetics by transforming challenges into opportunities. *Journal of the American Dietetic Association*, 1989;89:1441–1443.

40. Calvert-Finn S, Bajus B. President's page: 1992–1993 annual report. *Journal of the American Dietetic Association*, 1993;93:1448–1451.

41. Vickery CE, Cotugna N. *Legends and Legacies*. Dubuque: Kendall/Hunt Publishing Co., 1990.

42. Hess MA. President's page: 1990–1991 annual report. *Journal of the American Dietetic Association*, 1992;92:94–98.

43. See Note 42, above.

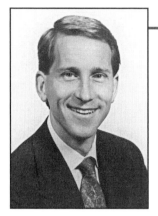

Marty Yadrick

Computrition, Inc.
Chatsworth, California

M y first exposure to dietetics as a career option was through my sister, Kathleen Yadrick, who is now an associate professor of dietetics at the University of Southern Mississippi. I have always looked up to and been proud of Kathy, and although my decision to enter the same profession was not necessarily to follow in her footsteps, her enthusiasm for and success in her career has always been an inspiration to me.

I first became interested in preventive medicine and how proper nutrition could help reduce the risk of disease. Because of this interest, I sought an internship that had a clinical emphasis and completed my dietetic internship at the University of Kansas Medical Center. My first job was as a long-term care dietitian at Truman Medical Center East in Kansas City, Missouri. In addition to being responsible for assessments and intervention for 200 patients, I gave lectures on geriatric nutrition to medical students. I next worked as a clinical dietitian at the Veterans Administration Medical Center in Leavenworth, Kansas, covering both acute and intermediate care patients. My next positions were at Research Medical Center as a cardiac rehabilitation dietitian and HealthPlus Wellness and Fitness Center as a sports/nutrition/wellness consultant.

During these years, I finished my master of science in dietetics and nutrition at the University of Kansas Medical Center, and my master of business administration at the University of Missouri–Kansas City. My interest in sports nutrition helped introduce me to the Sports, Cardiovascular, and Wellness Nutritionists practice group (SCAN) of the ADA. The members and leaders of SCAN have a contagious enthusiasm that has been extremely motivating for me in my career.

After completing my M.B.A., I worked as an administrative officer for the Department of Dietetics and Nutrition at the University of Kansas Medical Center. I served as financial officer for the department as well as assistant to the department chairman.

In my current position as training consultant for Computrition, Inc., I travel around the United States training customers on the use of our NutraCOM diet office automation software. In addition, I have been working for more than a year on the design of a new nutrition/risk assessment module. This project has been exciting for me, since it allows me to combine my clinical background with computer technology.

What I enjoy most about the field of nutrition is that it is so diverse, with career options limited only by the practitioner's imagination. Dietitians must continue to spread the word about good nutrition via the media, which will raise awareness of both our expertise and the potential healthcare cost savings which result from our intervention.

CHAPTER 2

Professionalism

What comes to mind when you hear someone described as professional? Responses to this question are generally varied and include such qualities as knowledgeable, ethical, caring, and well groomed. *Professionalism*, as defined by Webster's, is "the conduct, aims, or qualities that characterize or mark a profession or a professional person."[1] Along with the title *professional* comes a defined set of expectations. It is not enough to attain the title; one must also be committed to a well-defined pattern of responsibilities and activities.

In this chapter, the "conduct, aims, and qualities" considered characteristic of the dietetics profession are examined. The importance of showing respect and concern for people, being knowledgeable and keeping current with the latest research in one's area of practice, adherence to the strictest ethical standards, and commitment to the profession are emphasized. The role of professional societies, the benefits of membership, and a description of a selection of societies in the field are also included.

A HELPING PROFESSION

By its very nature, dietetics is a helping profession (Figure 2.1). Dietetic practice involves service to people.[2] The way this service is delivered is critically important. Respect, caring, and concern for people and their value systems are basic to the concept of professionalism. These characteristics may be manifested in many ways, not the least of which is respect for the dignity of each and every person. An understanding of individual differences—such as gender, ethnicity, and religion—is also critical for effective practice.

THE CHALLENGE AND REWARD OF LIFETIME LEARNING

Professional competence in the dietetic profession is ensured by the autonomous accrediting body of the ADA, the Commission on Dietetic Registration. It requires that practitioners complete an approved or accredited educational program and then maintain

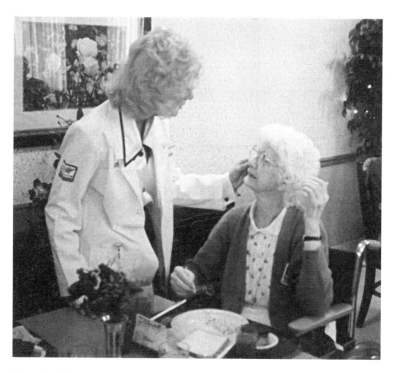

Figure 2.1
A dietary manager and one of her health center's residents.

competence through a system of continuing education. This continuing education may take the form of journal or textbook reading or attending and participating in seminars, conferences (Figure 2.2), meetings, exhibits, and college courses. Because the field of nutrition is so dynamic, the form and content of the continuing education should be carefully chosen to enhance the quality of the professional's practice.

Goals of Lifetime Education for the Dietetic Practitioner

Dietetic Practitioners:

1. *Are committed to excellence in the nutritional care of individuals and groups.* All dietetic practitioners contribute to nutritional care. Dietetic practitioners are dedicated to excellence in professional service. In the pursuit of excellence, they are responsible for the establishment of goals and the assessment of progress towards these goals.

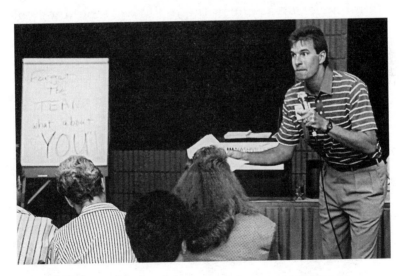

Figure 2.2
Dietary managers listen to a speaker at their annual meeting.
Source: Photo courtesy of the Dietary Managers Association.

2. *Comprehend, interpret, and apply the science and art of nutrition in the promotion of individual, group, and community health.* Dietetic practitioners need a thorough knowledge of the scientific bases of human nutritional needs, including biochemical, physiological, and psychological relationships throughout life, in health and disease. Interpretation and application of the science of nutrition requires creativity in dealing with people and situations, knowledge of food in its many implications for health, and the ability to communicate directly to people or indirectly through the efforts of others for nutritional care.

3. *Understand the significance of scientific inquiry and interpretation in advancing professional knowledge and improving standards of performance.* It is essential for dietitians to understand and appreciate research, and to be able to evaluate and interpret findings. The scope of dietetic research is broad. It includes such areas as nutritional (Figure 2.3), behavioral (Figure 2.4), and managerial sciences (Figure 2.5); technological developments in food production (Figures 2.6 and 2.7), processing, and marketing; foodservice systems and equipment; and information processing. The dietetic practitioner evaluates new research findings and utilizes those that are valid and appropriate for the nutritional care of people.

4. *Share responsibility with associated professionals by contributing specialized knowledge of nutrition.* Dietetic practitioners collaborate with others in planning, executing, and evaluating comprehensive healthcare programs. The prevention, treatment, and control of health problems of individuals, families, groups, or communities often have a nutritional component. This care may be given in a variety of settings: hospitals, extended-care facilities, government or voluntary health agencies, industries, businesses, or schools.

5. *Adapt planning and performance to environmental factors, recognizing physiological, psychological, social, political, cultural, and economic influences.* Dietetic practitioners are alert to emerging concepts in science and technology, and the envi-

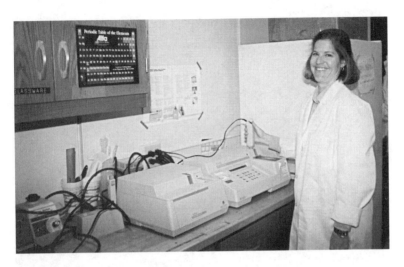

Figure 2.3
A research dietitian at work on a chemical panel analyzer.

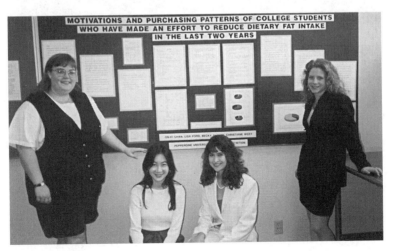

Figure 2.4
Dietetic students displaying their undergraduate research project.

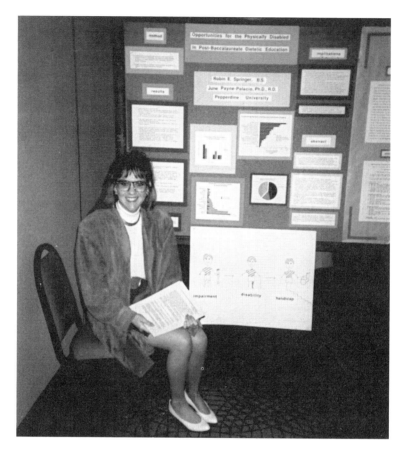

Figure 2.5
An undergraduate dietetics student displays her research
project at a professional meeting.

ronmental influences within society which will
require alteration in order to achieve them. They
are prepared to accept and work with individual
differences in food practices and varying attitudes
toward the role of nutrition in the promotion of
health and the control of disease.

6. *Demonstrate respect and empathy for people and
an appreciation of the individual's capacity to
change and develop.* Sensitivity to and acceptance
of the attitudes and behavior of individuals is
essential for teaching, guiding, and directing.

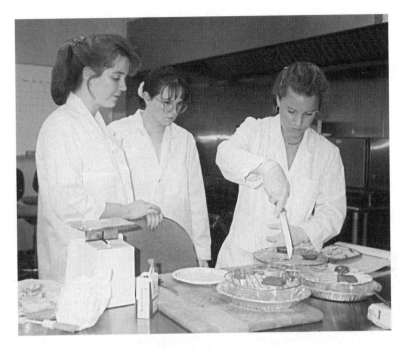

Figure 2.6
Dietetics students learn methods of food production.

Dietetic practitioners are responsible for providing an atmosphere in which an individual may be motivated to learn. When the teacher and the learner are mutually involved, both become better and more responsive individuals.

7. *Are competent in managing available resources in the provision of nutritional care.* Management is the coordination of available resources to achieve specified goals. Managerial competency is essential for all dietetic practitioners. The provision of nutritional care requires effective management of resources—physical facilities, finances, and people—so that people needing care receive it. New management theories and the evolution of health care emphasize the need for anticipatory management.

Dietetic practitioners recognize that one of their most important resources is themselves. Compe-

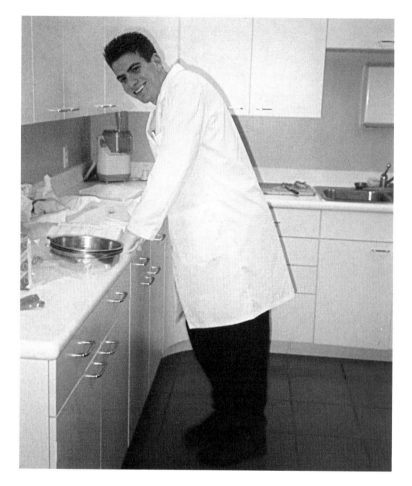

Figure 2.7
A dietetic student in a food science lab.

tency in management includes ability to assess and use one's own time and talents effectively.

8. *Manifest proficiency in communication.* Skill in communicating necessitates effective listening, speaking, reading, and writing. Dietetic practitioners, with an awareness of modern communication theory and methods, select the channels through which they can best communicate.

9. *Maintain the discipline and self-awareness of the professional and accept responsibility for their continuing professional development.* Recognition of the meaning of being professional—through self-appraisal, self-discipline, and continuing education—is essential for the dietetic practitioner. Planning for excellence necessitates formulating short- and long-term goals for professional development. Personal motivation, initiative, resourcefulness, and judgment need to be continuously exercised by the dietetic practitioner.

Receptiveness to new experiences and the pursuit of scientific inquiry are integral to continuing development. With increasing breadth of experience comes increased self-confidence and potential. These attributes, together with increasing flexibility, will contribute immeasurably to a lifetime of creative productivity.[3]

PROFESSIONAL ETHICS

Ethical issues faced by members of the dietetics profession are as diverse as the settings in which members practice. In medical and clinical settings, patients' rights, confidentiality of information, and the provision of food and water are the primary issues that must be confronted. In foodservice settings, ethical issues revolve around the management of money, personnel, materials, and time. In research and education, issues of plagiarism and research design involving animals or human beings are issues of ethical concern.[4]

Every professional association must address the issue of acceptable professional behavior. This is usually accomplished through a written document called a code of ethics. The code describes the philosophy and expectations of conduct to which the association agrees its members should adhere. The following is an example of one such code of ethics, developed by The American Dietetic Association in 1987.

Code of Ethics for the Profession of Dietetics

Preamble

The American Dietetic Association and its credentialing agency, the Commission on Dietetic Registration, believe it is in the best interests of the profession and the public it serves that a *Code of Ethics* provide guidance to dietetic practitioners in their professional practice and conduct. Dietetic practitioners have voluntarily developed a *Code of Ethics* to reflect the ethical principles guiding the dietetic profession and to outline commitments and obligations of the dietetic practitioner to self, client, society, and the profession.

The purpose of the Commission on Dietetic Registration is to assist in protecting the nutritional health, safety, and welfare of the public by establishing and enforcing qualifications for dietetic registration and for issuing voluntary credentials to individuals who have attained those qualifications. The Commission has adopted this *Code* to apply to individuals who hold these credentials.

The Ethics Code applies in its entirety to members of The American Dietetic Association who are Registered Dietitians (R.D.s) or Dietetic Technicians, Registered (D.T.R.s). Except for sections solely dealing with the credential, the *Code* applies to all American Dietetic Association members who are not R.D.s or D.T.R.s. Except for aspects solely dealing with membership, the *Code* applies to all R.D.s and D.T.R.s who are not ADA members. All of the aforementioned are referred to in the *Code* as "dietetic practitioners."

Principles

1. The dietetic practitioner provides professional services with objectivity and with respect for the unique needs and values of individuals.

2. The dietetic practitioner avoids discrimination against other individuals on the basis of race, creed, religion, sex, age, and national origin.

3. The dietetic practitioner fulfills professional commitments in good faith.

4. The dietetic practitioner conducts him/herself with honesty, integrity, and fairness.

5. The dietetic practitioner remains free of conflict of interest, while fulfilling the objectives and maintaining the integrity of the dietetic profession.

6. The dietetic practitioner maintains confidentiality of information.

7. The dietetic practitioner practices dietetics based on scientific principles and current information.

8. The dietetic practitioner assumes responsibility and accountability for personal competence in practice.

9. The dietetic practitioner recognizes and exercises professional judgment within the limits of his/her qualifications and seeks counsel or makes referrals as appropriate.

10. The dietetic practitioner provides sufficient information to enable clients to make their own informed decisions.

11. The dietetic practitioner who wishes to inform the public and colleagues of his/her services does so by using factual information. The dietetic practitioner does not advertise in a false or misleading manner.

12. The dietetic practitioner promotes or endorses products in a manner that is neither false or misleading.

13. The dietetic practitioner permits use of his/her name for the purpose of certifying that dietetic services have been rendered only if he/she has provided or supervised the provision of those services.

14. The dietetic practitioner accurately presents professional qualifications and credentials.

    a. The dietetic practitioner uses "R.D." or "registered dietitian" and "D.T.R." or "dietetic technician, registered" only when registration is current and authorized by the Commission on Dietetic Registration.

    b. The dietetic practitioner provides accurate information and complies with all requirements of the Commission on Dietetic Registration program in which he/she is seeking initial or continued credentials from the Commission on Dietetic Registration.

    c. The dietetic practitioner is subject to disciplinary action for aiding another person in violating any

Commission on Dietetic Registration requirements or aiding another person in representing himself/herself as an R.D. or D.T.R. when he/she is not.

15. The dietetic practitioner presents substantiated information and interprets controversial information without personal bias, recognizing that legitimate differences of opinion exist.

16. The dietetic practitioner makes all reasonable effort to avoid bias in any kind of professional evaluation. The dietetic practitioner provides objective evaluation of candidates for professional association membership, awards, scholarships, or job advancements.

17. The dietetic practitioner voluntarily withdraws from professional practice under the following circumstances:

   a. The dietetic practitioner has engaged in any substance abuse that could affect his/her practice.

   b. The dietetic practitioner has been adjudged by a court to be mentally incompetent.

   c. The dietetic practitioner has an emotional or mental disability that affects his/her practice in a manner that could harm the client.

18. The dietetic practitioner complies with all applicable laws and regulations concerning the profession. The dietetic practitioner is subject to disciplinary action under the following circumstances:

   a. The dietetic practitioner has been convicted of a crime under the laws of the United States which is a felony or a misdemeanor, an essential element of which is dishonesty and which is related to the practice of the profession.

   b. The dietetic practitioner has been disciplined by a state, and at least one of the grounds for the discipline is the same or substantially equivalent to these principles.

   c. The dietetic practitioner has committed an act of misfeasance or malfeasance which is directly related to the practice of the profession as determined by a court of competent jurisdiction, a licensing board, or an agency of a governmental body.

19. The dietetic practitioner accepts the obligation to protect society and the profession by upholding the *Code of Ethics for the Profession of Dietetics* and by reporting alleged violations of the *Code* through the defined review process of The American Dietetic Association and its credentialing agency, the Commission on Dietetic Registration.[5]

Purpose of a Code of Ethics

The purpose of a professional code of ethics is to reflect the principles of the profession and to provide an outline of the obligations of the member of that profession to self, client, society, and the profession. The *Code of Ethics for the Profession of Dietetics* addresses the provision of professional services, the accurate presentation of credentials and qualifications, standards for avoiding conflict of interest, and accountability for professional competence in practice. The *Code* also speaks to compliance with laws and regulations concerning the profession, presentation of substantiated information, confidentiality of information, the honesty, integrity and fairness of the member, and the obligation to uphold the standards of the profession by reporting apparent violations.[6]

New members joining the ADA receive a copy of the code and sign a statement stating they will abide by it. A study conducted recently found that the majority of dietitians agree with and adhere to the *Code*.[7] The review process for violations of this code includes a review of the complaint, an investigation, a hearing, and, finally, a decision and recommendation. The alleged respondent may be acquitted or, if found guilty, censored, temporarily suspended, or expelled from membership.

COMMITMENT TO THE PROFESSION

Those demonstrating professionalism in dietetic practice have a sense of commitment to the growth of the profession, both as a field of intellectual endeavor and as a society where people of similar purpose band together.[8] This commitment is best demonstrated by active participation in a professional association. Professional associations rely heavily on the work of volunteers at all levels—local, state, and national (Figure 2.8). It is through this collective energy of many professionals working together that an association becomes dynamic and productive. As Peter Drucker has said, "No organization can do better than the people it has."[9]

The benefits of professional association membership are both tangible and intangible. The tangible benefits may include receipt of publications, continuing education opportunities, lobbying on key legislative issues, public relations and marketing efforts, public recognition of professional achievements, student scholarship programs, member loan programs, discounts on rental cars and publications, travel programs, association-sponsored credit cards, group-rate medical and life insurance, and professional liability insurance, to mention just a few.

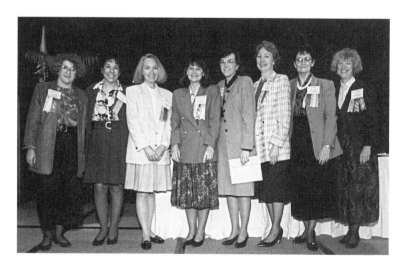

Figure 2.8
The executive board of a state dietetic association.

Of even greater importance are the intangible benefits that accrue from professional association involvement. The friendships that develop, the professional contacts that are made, the opportunity to develop leadership skills, the sense of creative stimulation, the excitement of being a part of the action, and the opportunity to impact issues and shape policy for the good of the profession are good reasons to volunteer at some level of commitment (Figures 2.9 and 2.10).

For students, there are additional advantages of active participation. Students have an opportunity to:

- develop skills in public speaking, writing, program planning and organizing;
- network with dietitians, technicians, and other students;
- observe professional role models; and

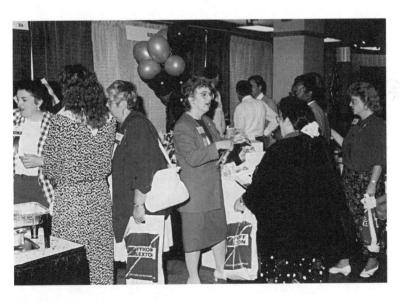

Figure 2.9
Dietary managers attend a foodservice products expo held in conjunction with their annual meeting.
Source: Photo courtesy of the Dietary Managers Association.

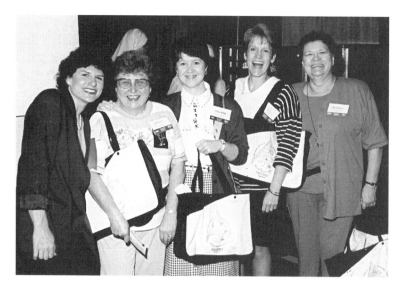

Figure 2.10
Camarderie is shared among dietary managers at their
annual meeting.
Source: Photo courtesy of the Dietary Managers Association.

- enhance visibility, for scholarships, internships, and
  future permanent employment.

The biggest risk one faces is the time commitment
required. Frustrations may also arise when costs exceed
the resources available for certain plans, or when members disagree. But these are minor considerations when
one considers the risk of *not* being involved.[10]

SELECTED PROFESSIONAL ASSOCIATIONS

The American Dietetic Association (ADA)

The nation's largest professional organization for food
and nutrition professionals was founded in 1917 and
now has approximately 63,000 members. There are a
number of categories of membership with varying educational requirements for eligibility; however, the
majority of members are dietitians or dietetic techni-

cians. Affiliated dietetic associations exist in every state and in Puerto Rico and Europe. The mission of the ADA is to serve the public through the promotion of optimal nutrition, health, and well-being. This association will be discussed in more detail in Chapter 3.

The Dietary Managers Association (DMA)

Founded in 1960, DMA is the national professional organization for dietary managers. Associate and student memberships are available. Total membership now exceeds 13,000. This association will be discussed in more detail in Chapter 4.

American Institute of Nutrition (AIN)

AIN is the principal professional organization of nutrition research scientists in the United States. With approximately 3,000 members from 40 countries, AIN was chartered by the Regents of the University of the State of New York in 1933. "Members are nominated by fellow scientists on the basis of demonstrated research competence and productivity in experimental nutrition or service to the discipline of nutrition." Graduate students who intend to pursue a career in nutrition research are eligible for membership. Those who have published meritorious original research in clinical nutrition are eligible for nomination for membership in the American Society for Clinical Nutrition (ASCN), the clinical division of AIN. ASCN publishes the *American Journal of Clinical Nutrition*. AIN is a corporate member of the Federation of American Societies of Experimental Biology (FASEB) and holds an annual meeting in conjunction with other FASEB societies. AIN publishes the monthly *Journal of Nutrition* and a quarterly newsletter, *Nutrition Notes*. AIN has an extensive awards and recognition program as well as a graduate research competition. It also publishes a graduate education directory.

American Society for Parenteral and Enteral Nutrition (ASPEN)

ASPEN's membership includes dietitians, nurses, physicians, pharmacists, and other health-care providers involved or interested in nutrition support of patients. Student membership is also available. The organization publishes the *Journal of Parenteral and Enteral Nutrition* and *Nutrition in Clinical Practice* on a bimonthly basis; establishes and publishes standards and clinical guidelines for nutrition support; organizes and sponsors an annual multidisciplinary nutrition conference; administers a specialty certification program for nurses and dietitians; provides a local chapter program; has awards and self-assessment programs; and serves as an advocate for nutrition support services.

Society of Nutrition Education (SNE)

Members in SNE, both in the student or regular category, are required to have at least two college-level courses in nutrition. The goal of the association is to enhance the ability of its members to help the public make informed food choices. Members are organized into practice divisions: communications, food and nutrition extension educators, higher education, international nutrition education, nutrition educators for children, nutrition educators with industry, public health nutrition, and sustainable food systems. A number of states have nutrition councils affiliated with SNE. The society publishes the *Journal of Nutrition Education* and the *SNE Communicator*.

National Restaurant Association (NRA)

Founded in 1919, the NRA's mission is to protect, promote, and educate the members of the foodservice industry. The NRA has 25,000 members representing more than 150,000 food-service operations. The benefits of membership include a monthly magazine,

Restaurants USA; a weekly legislative report, *Washington Weekly*; research reports; educational seminars and materials; promotion of the industry to the government and the public; access to mailing lists and referrals; and annual shows. Membership is open to foodservice operators, businesses that provide products and services to the industry, students, and faculty. Dues are based on type of membership and annual gross sales of the business. Dietetic practitioners involved in foodservice management or sales and marketing of foodservice products find membership in NRA beneficial.

American Home Economics Association (AHEA)

One of the oldest professional organizations of all, AHEA was founded in 1909 as a scientific and educational society. Its founder, Ellen Richards, attended the Lake Placid Conference and was instrumental in changing the name of the discipline from domestic science to home economics. Now, with nearly 20,000 members, its purpose is to improve the quality and standards of individual and family life through education, research, cooperative programs, and public information. Membership includes educators, lecturers, school administrators, extension home economists, counselors, child-care workers, dietitians, consultants, product development specialists, public relations directors, homemakers, and researchers. AHEA publishes the *Journal of Home Economics* and the *Home Economics Research Journal*. Each state has an affiliate association that sponsors meetings and programs throughout the year. The national association puts on an annual meeting and exposition.

National Association of Food Equipment Manufacturers (NAFEM)

NAFEM's active membership is made up of commercial foodservice equipment and supplies manufacturers representing more than 600 companies in the United States and Canada. Industry trade publications are associate members of NAFEM. Founded in 1948, NAFEM's mission is to develop and promote cooperative programs and activities that will improve the level of professionalism and broaden knowledge within the foodservice equipment and supplies industry. Dietetic practitioners involved in layout and design consulting, and those in sales and marketing of foodservice equipment, find membership in NAFEM beneficial.

American School Food Service Association (ASFSA)

ASFSA was founded in 1946, the same year that the National School Lunch Act became law. Its mission is to protect and enhance children's health and well-being by operating nutritious foodservice programs and providing proper nutrition education in public and nonprofit private schools. Of more than 65,000 members, nearly 32,000 are certified through a program that requires the completion of coursework in sanitation, safety, technical skills, management, and nutrition. ASFSA publishes the *School Food Service Journal*, a monthly magazine, and the *School Food Service Research Review*, a semiannual journal. ASFSA has lobbied for legislation involving child nutrition policies and programs. The ASFSA sponsors a number of meetings and conferences throughout the year, including an annual conference and exhibition.

Foodservice Consultants Society International (FCSI)

FCSI has members in 30 countries. It publishes a quarterly journal, *The Consultant*; a member newsletter, *The Spec Sheet*; a membership directory; a products-buying guide; a bulletin, *FCSI/Tech*; and *Critical MAS*, a newsletter of case studies, opinions, and trends. To qualify for professional membership in FCSI, one must have at least ten years experience as a foodservice consultant, four years of college, have been a project director for five years, be qualified to design and implement foodservice programs, be employed as a professional consultant, and submit an article of at least 2,000 words for publication in *The Consultant.* Other categories of membership, like student member, have less-strict requirements.

National Association of College and University Food Services (NACUFS)

The mission of NACUFS is to promote the highest quality of food service on school, college, and university campuses by providing educational and training opportunities, technical assistance, related industry information and support for research to the membership. The members of NACUFS are campus foodservice directors and support staff from over 540 colleges and universities in the United States, Canada, and abroad. NACUFS supports students with a summer internship program, scholarships, and awards. Benefits to members include networking opportunities from attending conferences, educational programs, and committee meetings; industry contacts; peer consultation services; educational and professional development programs; provision of comparative statistics; job placement; publications; professional recognition; and leadership opportunities.

SUMMARY

"A profession is shaped and molded by dynamic and dedicated individuals whose careers have made a difference."[11] The profession of dietetics requires a team approach with each member of the team the very embodiment of professionalism: knowledgeable, caring, concerned, respectful, ethical, committed to the profession, and active in the professional organization. The dietetic team member has an essential orientation to the interest of others—the patient, the client, the community, etc. The dietetic team member is unquestionably ethical in all matters. The dietetic team member is committed to preserving the credibility and dignity of the profession and believes that the practice of dietetics has an impact on the quality of life of others. Putting aside personal benefits and risks, the dietetic team member recognizes the importance of professional association involvement for the good of the profession as a whole.

SUGGESTED ACTIVITIES

1. Visit your school library to determine which nutrition periodicals are available. Carefully examine at least one issue of each and write one or two sentences describing the journal. For example, one publication might be described as "a monthly publication with literature reviews of nutrition research and occasional book reviews. Frequently, many articles in an issue are related to the same topic."

2. Carefully examine an issue of a popular magazine that contains articles on nutrition, such as *Shape* or *Hippocrates*. Briefly evaluate the reliability and validity of the nutrition content.

3. Attend a continuing education program sponsored by a local dietetic association. Write a report describing what is required of attendees in order to obtain continuing education credit.

4. Set some goals for professional development and self-improvement. Assign top priority to three and describe why you chose these three.

5. Discuss the following scenario: A private practice dietitian regularly recommends that clients take megadoses of several vitamins. The dietitian bases the recommendation on years of research by a scientist who has testimonial evidence that the treatment works for a number of medical conditions. The dietitian's clients claim to have been helped

when traditional medicine has failed. Has a code of ethics been violated? What are the issues here?

NOTES

1. Gove PB, ed. *Webster's Third New International Dictionary.* Springfield, MA: G & C Merriam Co., 1971.

2. Combs AW, Avila DL, Purkey WW. *Helping Relationships: Basic Concepts for the Helping Professions.* Boston: Allyn and Bacon, Inc., 1976.

3. Committee on Goals of Education for Dietetics, Dietetic Internship Council, The American Dietetic Association. Goals of lifetime education of the dietitian. *Journal of the American Dietetic Association,* 1969;54:91–93.

4. Neville JN, Chernoff R. President's page: Professional ethics—everyone's issue. *Journal of the American Dietetic Association,* 1988;88: 1285–1287.

5. American Dietetic Association. "Code of Ethics for the Profession of Dietetics." *Journal of the American Dietetic Association,* 1988;88 1592–1593.

6. Ethics Resources. Chicago: American Dietetic Association, August 1986.

7. Anderson SL. "Dietitians' practices and attitudes regarding the Code of Ethics for the Profession of Dietetics." *Journal of the American Dietetic Association,* 1993; 88–91.

8. Mason M, Wenberg BG, and Welsh PK. *The Dynamics of Clinical Dietetics,* 2d ed. New York: John Wiley & Sons, Inc., 1982.

9. Drucker PF. *Managing the Nonprofit Organization.* New York: Harper Collins, 1990.

10. Dodd JL. "President's page: The benefits and risks of membership." *Journal of the American Dietetic Association,* 1992;92:362.

11. Vickery CE, Cotugna N. *Legends and Legacies*. Dubuque: Kendall/Hunt Publishing Co., 1990.

SELECTED RESOURCES

American Dietetic Association
216 West Jackson Blvd., Suite 800
Chicago, IL 60606–6995
312–899–0040

Dietary Managers Association
One Pierce Place, Suite 1220W
Itasca, IL 60143–3111
708–775–9200 or FAX 708–775–9250

National Association of Food Equipment Manufacturers
401 N. Michigan Avenue
Chicago, IL 60611–4267
312–644–6610 or FAX 312–245–1080

American Home Economics Association
1555 King Street
Alexandria, VA 22314
703–706–4600 or FAX 703–706–HOME

Foodservice Consultants Society International
304 West Liberty Street, Suite 201
Louisville, KY 40202
502–583–3783

American School Food Service Association
1600 Duke Street, 7th Floor
Alexandria, VA 22314–3436
800–877–8822 or FAX 703–739–3915

Society for Nutrition Education
2001 Killebrew Drive, Suite 340
Minneapolis, MN 55425–1882
612–854–0035 or FAX 612–854–7869

American Institute of Nutrition & The American Society for Clinical Nutrition, Inc.

9650 Rockville Pike
Bethesda, MD 20814–3998
AIN: 301–530–7050 ASCN: 301–530–7110 or FAX:
  301–571–1892

National Association of College and University Food
  Services
1405 South Harrison Road, Suite 303
Manly Miles Building, Michigan State University
East Lansing, MI 48824
517–332–2494 or FAX 517–332–8144

American Society for Parenteral and Enteral Nutrition
8630 Fenton Street, Suite 412
Silver Spring, MD 20910
301–587–6315

National Restaurant Association
1200 Seventeenth Street, NW
Washington, DC 20036–3097
202–331–5900

Food and Nutrition Information Center
National Agricultural Library, Room 304
Beltsville, MD 20705
301–344–3719

The National Dairy Council
6300 North River Road
Rosemont, IL 60018–4233
708–696–1020

American Council on Science and Health
1995 Broadway, 16th Floor
New York, NY 10023–5860
212–362–7044

Department of Agriculture, Human Nutrition Information Service
Federal Building
Hyattsville, MD 20782
301–436–8617

Food and Nutrition Program
American Medical Association
535 North Dearborn Street
Chicago, IL 60610
312–645–5000

National Institutes of Health
Bethesda, MD 20705
301–496–4000

ILSI/The Nutrition Foundation
1126 Sixteenth Street, NW
Washington, DC 20036
202–857–3680

Institute of Food Technologists
221 North LaSalle Street
Chicago, IL 60601
312–782–8424

Office of Disease Prevention and Health Promotion
National Health Information Center
P.O. Box 1133
Washington, DC 20013–1133
800–336–4797 or 301–565–4167 (in Maryland)

Consumer Information Center
Pueblo, CO 81009

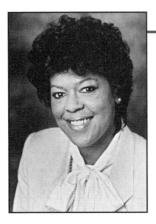

Bettye Nowlin

*Dairy Council of California
Culver City, California*

M y discovery of dietetics was completely accidental. At the end of my first year of college, I worked in the dietary department of our local hospital for the summer. It was there that I met the dietitian and learned more about the possibilities within the profession. Having the opportunity to gain experience in many different areas of dietetics during that summer really confirmed in my mind that this was what I wanted to do.

Upon returning to school at Tennessee Agricultural and Industrial University in Nashville, I completed requirements for two degrees: one in foods and nutrition and one in home economics education with a teaching credential. After graduation, I accepted a dietetic internship at St. Luke's Hospital and Medical Center in New York City. I became a registered dietitian in 1969, when registration was first instituted. I later obtained a master's in public health nutrition (MPH) from the University of California at Los Angeles.

During my career, I have held all kinds of positions, including therapeutic dietitian at Cook County Hospital, administrative dietitian at Michael Reese Hospital and Medical Center, high school home economics teacher, and public health nutritionist, all in Chicago, Illinois. I then moved to Los Angeles, where I became involved as a nutrition consultant with Head Start and the Senior Feeding Programs. I also worked as nutrition education consultant, program director, and now manager of public affairs for the Dairy Council of California.

In my current position, I am responsible for developing and implementing a three-hour continuing education course for registered dietitians on counseling skills and behavior change theory. Workshops are conducted both in and outside of California. I also am involved in developing partnerships and joint efforts on nutrition projects with other groups, and for strategic planning on nutrition issues that impact my area of responsibility.

Being involved in my profession has always been a priority. Some of my involvement includes being selected as one of the 16 original Ambassadors for the ADA. I have also served three years as a Director-at-Large on the ADA's Board of Directors and as a member of the national nominating committee. State and local dietetic association experiences have given me valuable experiences. These involvements have contributed much to my personal and professional development.

I would encourage students to become involved in the Student Dietetic Association at their university and to volunteer for activities within their local dietetic association. Attending local, state, and national dietetics meetings are a wonderful way to network and learn more about the profession. Volunteering for roles is mutually beneficial, as it helps build leadership skills and confidence. After several years of volunteering, I have been awarded the California Dietetic Association's Distinguished Service Award, the Excellence in Community Nutrition Award, and ADA's Medallion Award.

Choosing dietetics as a career has allowed me to do the things that give me pleasure and satisfaction and to work and interact with colleagues that I care about. This is an honor in itself.

CHAPTER 3

The American Dietetic Association

The American Dietetic Association (ADA) is the largest association of nutrition professionals in the world.[1] Founded in Cleveland, Ohio, in 1917, the Association has grown to almost 66,000 members.[2] The purpose of this chapter is to help you understand the mission, vision, and values of the Association and to become knowledgeable about the structure and organization of the Association and its headquarters office.

WHO ARE THE MEMBERS OF ADA?

There are five classifications of membership in the ADA: active, associate, retired, returning student, and honorary.[3] You may utilize several of these membership categories as you move through your professional life.

There are four types of individuals who may apply for the active member classification. First, **active members** include any person who has a bachelor's degree from a regionally accredited college or university or its equivalent, meets academic requirements specified by ADA, and meets one or more of the following criteria:

1. is a Registered Dietitian, credentialed by the Commission on Dietetic Registration,

2. has completed a supervised practice program accredited/approved by the Commission on Accreditation/Approval for Dietetics Education (CAADE),

3. has earned a master's or doctoral degree conferred by a regionally accredited college or university.

Second, any person may apply for actual membership who has earned a master's or doctoral degree or equivalent, and who holds one degree (baccalaureate, master's, doctoral) in one of the following areas: dietetics, foods and nutrition, nutrition, community/public health nutrition, food science, or foodservice systems management. Each degree must be conferred by a regionally accredited college or university.

Third, any person who meets one or more of the following criteria may apply for active membership:

1. is a Dietetic Technician, Registered (D.T.R.) credentialed by the Commission on Dietetic Registration or has established eligibility to write the examination for dietetic technicians.

2. has completed an associate degree program for dietetic technicians that has been accredited/approved by CAADE.

3. is a graduate of a baccalaureate degree program and meets academic requirements specified by ADA, with CAADE-approved dietetic technician program experience.

Finally, any person who has paid the optional one-time dues to obtain life membership in the Association, or has completed a term as president of the Association may be an active member.

Associate members include any person who meets one of the following criteria and is not eligible for active membership:

1. is a graduate of a baccalaureate degree program and meets requirements specified by ADA.

2. is an undergraduate or associate degree student enrolled in a CAADE-accredited/approved dietetic program, or is a graduate student meeting the minimum academic requirements in a CAADE-approved/accredited program.
3. is a student enrolled in a supervised practice program accredited/approved by CAADE.
4. is a student in a regionally accredited, postsecondary education program which is non-CAADE accredited/approved. This classification is available for three years to students who state intent to enter a CAADE-accredited/approved program.

See your dietetics program director for associate member information or call (800) 877–1600 for membership information. Joining ADA as a student is an excellent way to learn about the profession of dietetics and become familiar with its publications, activities, etc.

Retired members include any member of ADA who is no longer employed in dietetic practice or education and is at least 62 years old or who is retired due to permanent disability.

The **returning student** category includes any active member returning to school on a full-time basis for a baccalaureate or graduate degree in a dietetic course of study. Membership in the returning student class can be held for a maximum of five years and must be renewed annually.

The **honorary member** category is a special honor awarded to an individual who has made a notable contribution to the field of nutrition and dietetics and has been invited to be an honorary member by the Board of Directors of the Association.

MISSION, VISION, PHILOSOPHY, AND VALUES

In the late 1980s, the ADA Board of Directors endorsed a mission statement which defines the purpose of the organization. The mission of the ADA is as follows:

> The American Dietetic Association is the advocate of the dietetics profession serving the public through the promotion of optimal nutrition, health, and well-being.[3]

The words *advocate*, *serving the public*, and *promotion* explain ADA's focus. The Association acts as an advocate for its members, striving to position the dietitian as a nutrition expert in the eyes of the public, the medical community, legislators, and other constituencies. The members of the Association serve the public in numerous ways, through the promotion of optimal nutrition and health.

The vision statement of the Association serves as a guide to the officers of the Association as they plan the programs and activities in which the organization will be involved. The vision statement helps members understand the role the Association hopes to assume in the future. The vision statement of the ADA is as follows:

> Members of The American Dietetic Association will shape the food choices and impact the nutritional status of the public.[3]

The philosophy statement of the ADA sets the tone of customer service, which should be paramount in all interactions between dietitians and their clientele. The philosophy of the ADA states:

> Members of The American Dietetic Association serve the profession best by serving the public first.[3]

The values of the Association serve as a guide to action and a statement of attributes toward which all dietitians should strive.

> The actions of The American Dietetic Association and its members reflect the following values:

Excellence in the identification, development and delivery of quality programs, services, and products.

Leadership in significant food, nutrition and related health issues.

Integrity in all professional and personal actions.

Respect for diverse viewpoints and individual differences.

Communication that is timely and effective.

Collaboration for action on critical issues.

Fiscal Responsibility in effectively providing and managing human and financial resources.

Action that is timely and strategic.[4]

ADA HEADQUARTERS

The headquarters of The American Dietetic Association (216 W. Jackson Blvd., Chicago, IL 60606–6995, (800)877–1600) house the full-time paid staff members who carry on the day-to-day business of the Association (Figure 3.1). There are currently 150 paid employees of the Association.[4] Employees work in assigned groups which serve to support different aspects of ADA's focus.

Also located in Chicago are the American Dietetic Association Foundation (ADAF), the National Center for Nutrition and Dietetics (NCND), and the offices of the Commission on Dietetic Registration (CDR).

The **American Dietetic Association Foundation** funds education initiatives that promote public nutrition, health, and well-being. The ADAF is considered to be a not-for-profit corporation and is the largest private grantor of scholarship and fellowship funds in the field of dietetics. Students in dietetics and related fields are encouraged to apply for ADAF scholarships. Applications are typically due the middle of February each year, with awards made for the following academic year. Dietetic education program directors receive information about these scholarships every fall.

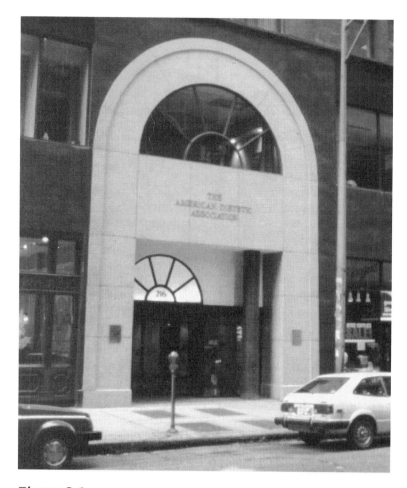

Figure 3.1
American Dietetic Association headquarters.

The **National Center for Nutrition and Dietetics** was established in 1990 as ADA's education center for the public. NCND contributes to ADA's mission of promoting optimal nutrition, health, and well-being through offering programs and services of interest to the public. These offerings include a toll-free Consumer Nutrition Hotline and RD referral service ((800)366–1655), staffed by a Registered Dietitian. This hotline allows consumers to hear prerecorded nutrition messages, speak to a Registered Dietitian, and obtain referrals to RDs in their area. The NCND also sponsors National Nutrition Month, which is celebrated each March under the theme "Eat Right America", and Project LEAN (Low-fat Eating for America Now).

The **Commission on Dietetic Registration** is the credentialing arm of the American Dietetic Association. CDR credentials individuals who have met its standards for competency to practice in the profession. The function of CDR is more fully discussed in Chapter 6.

The ADA also retains paid employees at an office in Washington, D.C. (1225 Eye Street, N.W., Suite 1250, Washington, DC 20005). These employees work on ADA's behalf on legislative matters which affect the future of the dietetics profession. Members may call the ADA Office of Government and Legal Affairs in Washington at (202)371–0500 if they have questions about legislative activities or issues affecting dietetics at the state or federal level.

THE VOLUNTEER ELEMENT OF ADA

The officers of the ADA are volunteers who are elected by the membership of the Association. Major offices are elected by national ballot; officers of the various subgroups (such as dietetic practice groups) are elected by members of that particular subgroup.

The work of the Association is accomplished by two major entities: the Board of Directors (BOD) and the House of Delegates (HOD).

The Board of Directors

The Board of Directors is responsible for the ADA's mission and vision and is the association's policy-making and governing body. The BOD manages the property and fiscal affairs of the Association, directs the implementation of approved actions, and monitors the outcomes of Association projects. The BOD comprises the following elected positions:

President (Chairman of the BOD)

President–Elect

Secretary/Treasurer

Secretary/Treasurer–Elect

Speaker of the House of Delegates

Speaker–Elect of the House of Delegates

President of the ADA Foundation

Chief Operating Officer

5 Directors–at–Large

2 Directors–at–Large Public Members (appointed by the BOD)

Chair of the Commission on Dietetic Registration (no vote)

Chair of the Commission on Accreditation/Approval for Dietetics Education (no vote)

The two commissions which are represented on the BOD are autonomous organizations, because of the nature of the business they conduct. These commissions direct accreditation of dietetic education programs and the credentialing of dietetics practitioners, two activities which must remain free from the influence of the Association. The Chairpersons of these two commissions sit on the BOD to facilitate communication between the commissions and the Association; however, they do not vote on issues which are brought before the BOD.

The BOD uses several committees to accomplish its work. These committees include the Board of Directors Executive Committee, the Budget and Fiscal Affairs Committee, the Legislative and Public Policy Committee, the Diversity Committee, and the Scholarship Committee.

The House of Delegates

The ADA House of Delegates is comparable to the United States House of Representatives. It provides a forum for membership and professional issues and establishes professional standards. Each state's dietetic association elects delegates to represent that state at the national level. The number of delegates a state has is based on the number of ADA members who live in that state. The House of Delegates has 138 members. The HOD is divided into 7 geographic areas, each with an Area Coordinator elected by national ballot. The Puerto Rico Dietetic Association has a representative in the HOD, as does the American European Dietetic Association, which represents American dietitians working in Europe.

State Affiliate Representatives in the ADA House of Delegates by Area

Area I	State	Number of Delegates
	Alaska	1
	California	9
	Hawaii	1
	Idaho	1
	Montana	1
	Oregon	2
	Washington	2
	Wyoming	1
	Total	20

Area II	State	Number of Delegates
	Iowa	2
	Michigan	3
	Minnesota	2
	Missouri	2
	Nebraska	1
	North Dakota	1
	South Dakota	1
	Wisconsin	3
	Total	17

Area III	State	Number of Delegates
	Alabama	2
	Arkansas	1
	Florida	4
	Georgia	2
	Louisiana	2
	Mississippi	1
	Puerto Rico	1
	South Carolina	1
	Total	*16*

Area IV	State	Number of Delegates
	Arizona	2
	Colorado	2
	Kansas	2
	Nevada	1
	New Mexico	1
	Oklahoma	2
	Texas	5
	Utah	1
	Total	*18*

Area V	State	Number of Delegates
	Illinois	4
	Indiana	2
	Kentucky	2
	Ohio	5
	Tennessee	2
	West Virginia	1
	Total	*18*

Area VI	State	Number of Delegates
	Delaware	1

	District of Columbia	1
	Maryland	2
	North Carolina	2
	Pennsylvania	5
	Virginia	2
	Total	*15*

Area VII	*State*	*Number of Delegates*
	Connecticut	2
	Maine	1
	Massachusetts	3
	New Hampshire	1
	New Jersey	3
	New York	7
	Rhode Island	1
	Vermont	1
	AEDA*	1
	Total	*22*

Members of the HOD are as follows:

Speaker (Chairman)

Speaker–Elect

7 Area Coordinators

15 Delegates who make up the Council on Professional Issues

    8 represent Dietetics Practice

    3 represent Dietetics Education

    3 represent Dietetics Research

    1 Dietetic Technician–at–Large

2 other Dietetic Technicians–at–Large

---

*American/European Dietetic Association.

112 Delegates representing state and affiliate dietetic associations listed above

The full HOD meets twice a year, immediately before the start of the annual meeting each fall and at the HOD Mid-Year Meeting, typically held at the end of April or beginning of May. Issues are discussed and debated both in area meetings and before the full HOD. Since delegates are the elected representatives of ADA members in their respective states, they bring to these discussions the views of their constituents back home. Observers are welcome to attend any of these sessions to gain a fuller appreciation of how the work of the Association is carried out. The formal HOD meeting, during which agenda items are voted on, is held on Sunday each time the HOD meets. It is a formal and impressive event.

STATE AFFILIATES AND DISTRICT DIETETIC ASSOCIATIONS

Each state and the District of Columbia has its own state dietetic association affiliated with The American Dietetic Association. When an individual joins The ADA, a percentage of their dues is rebated to the state where they live, automatically making them a member of their state dietetics association. State dietetic associations elect their own officers and host their own meetings once or twice a year.

Each state association comprises district dietetic associations that serve the needs of dietitians in specific areas within the state. There are currently approximately 220 district associations in the United States. District associations may comprise a single metropolitan area or several counties. Membership in district associations is *not* automatic. These groups receive no rebates from the national level and typically charge a separate membership fee to support their programming efforts.

Involvement in district and state dietetic associations is a great way for new dietetics graduates to become involved in a professional organization. Opportunities for leadership development and personal/professional growth abound in these groups.

DIETETIC PRACTICE GROUPS

Dietetic practice groups (DPGs) comprise individuals who have a common interest in a particular area of dietetics practice, regardless of membership classification or employment status. A dietetic practice group may be formed when at least 300 members petition the House of Delegates Council on Professional Issues to form such a group.

DPGs are national in scope and have their own elected officers and dues. These groups engage in activities which meet the needs of their members, such as producing newsletters or providing continuing education events. These groups provide members the opportunity to develop leadership skills through participation on committees or through appointment or election to offices.

Following is a list of the current DPGs of The American Dietetic Association:

Division of Community Nutrition
  Public Health Nutrition
  Gerontological Nutritionists
  Dietetics in Development and Psychiatric Disorders
  Vegetarian Nutrition
  Hunger and Malnutrition
Division of Clinical Nutrition
  Oncology Nutrition
  Renal Dietitians
  Pediatric Nutrition
  Diabetes Care and Education
  Dietitians in Nutrition Support
  Dietetics in Physical Medicine and Rehabilitation
  Dietitians in General Clinical Practice

Division of Consultation and Business Practice
  Consulting Nutritionists
  Consultant Dietitians in Health-Care Facilities
  Dietitians in Business and Communications
  Sports, Cardiovascular, and Wellness Nutritionists
Division of Food and Nutrition Management
  Management in Health-Care Systems
  School Nutrition Services
  Clinical Nutrition Management
  Technical Practice in Dietetics
Division of Education and Research
  Dietetic Educators of Practitioners
  Nutrition Educators of Health Professionals
  Nutrition Education for the Public
  Nutrition Research

WHY SHOULD I BE A MEMBER OF THE AMERICAN DIETETIC ASSOCIATION?

Membership in a professional association is a privilege. Professional associations like the ADA provide opportunities for personal and professional growth, leadership, and lasting friendships. Whereas one dietitian alone may not feel that he or she can make a difference, the strength of 66,000 dietitians can make their voices heard in setting public policy or influencing public opinion. The ADA plays a key role in influencing issues such as health-care reform, food labeling, child nutrition programs, nutrition screening for the elderly, and long-term care. The ADA provides expert testimony at Congressional hearings and comments on proposed federal and state legislation. The Association also publishes position papers, which outline ADA's stand on a variety of timely, and sometimes controversial, topics.

The ADA also conducts a number of important programs, campaigns, and other outreach efforts, to promote health and well-being and to position Registered Dietitians as nutrition experts. Some examples include:

- *The Nutrition and Health Campaign for Women.* This campaign educates women about the impact of nutrition on their health. It promotes research into links between nutrition and healthy weight and heart disease, breast cancer, osteoporosis and diabetes.
- *The Physician Nutrition Education Project.* This program is designed to help physicians maintain their awareness of comprehensive health care and the role of the dietitian as a nutrition expert.
- *The Nationwide Nutrition Network.* This network helps consumers, physicians, and businesses find Registered Dietitians in their communities who can provide services in the management of weight, meal planning, sports nutrition, cardiovascular disease, HIV/AIDS, and diabetes, among other topics.
- *The Child Nutrition and Health Campaign.* This consumer education campaign utilizes a nationally recognized panel of child nutrition experts to report on the nutrition needs of children and help educate consumers—especially parents, those who work with children, and the media.

SUMMARY

Belonging to the American Dietetic Association, your state and district dietetic associations, and the ADA dietetic practice groups can enhance and enrich your professional and personal growth. Communication, networking, leadership opportunities, and other member benefits are available to those who participate. You determine your own level of involvement, and, thus, your own level of satisfaction. Become actively involved in the ADA and reap the rewards of an active and involved professional life.

SUGGESTED ACTIVITIES

1. Attend a district, state, or national dietetics meeting.
2. Look for the issue of the *ADA Journal* that showcases the new officers of the Association. Read the brief description about each person and find out in what area of dietetics each person works.
3. Invite the delegate(s) to ADA's House of Delegates from your state to your class to talk about current issues relevant to dietetics.
4. Does your school have a Student Dietetic Association (SDA)? If so, do you actively participate? If not, attend the next meeting and find out what is going on. If your school does not have a Student Dietetic Association, get together with your classmates and form such an association. Contact other schools that have dietetics programs to find out if they have an SDA and what types of activities they sponsor.

NOTES

1. *The American Dietetic Association: Promoting Better Health Through Better Nutrition.* Chicago: The American Dietetic Association; 1995.
2. Cassell JA. *Carry the Flame: The History of The American Dietetic Association.* Chicago: The American Dietetic Association; 1990. American Dietetic Association, Membership Committee, House of Delegates Mid-Year Meeting Report; April, 1995.
3. Bylaws of The American Dietetic Association. Passed by the House of Delegates, April 30, 1995, Oak Brook, Illinois.
4. Lechowich K. Personal communication, 11 May, 1995.

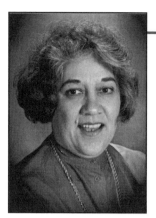

Cheryl Bittle

*Portland Area Indian
Health Service
Portland, Oregon*

I am a native of Oklahoma and a member of the Creek
Indian Tribe. After finishing a degree in Foods, Nutrition,
and Institutional Administration at Oklahoma State University,
I completed a dietetic internship at Yale–New Haven Hospital
in New Haven, Connecticut. Further education included a
master's degree in public health nutrition at Case Western
Reserve University in Cleveland and a Ph.D. in nutrition, food
science, and organizational management from the University
of Tennessee, Knoxville.

My background in dietetics has afforded me the opportunity to work in a variety of settings. I have worked as a dietitian in hospitals in West Virginia and Illinois, as a public
health nutritionist at the Comanche County (Oklahoma)
Health Department, as a nutrition consultant with maternal
and child health programs in Oklahoma, and as an assistant
professor at Oregon State University.

My current position is with the Portland Area Indian Health
Service as director, office of health programs. This position
involves the supervision of area health specialists in areas
such as laboratory/radiology, maternal and child health,
health education, dental services, nutrition and dietetics,
clinic and community nursing, pharmacy, mental health, and
social services. As a member of the executive staff, I am
involved in a variety of activities related to tribal self-gover-
nance, clinical development, and expansion of community-

based health services over the states of Oregon, Washington, and Idaho.

Participation in professional organizations is very important to me. I am involved in the American Dietetic Association, the Oregon Dietetic Association, the American Public Health Association, and the Society of Nutrition Education. I have been fortunate to hold offices in each of these groups. One of the highlights of my involvement was the opportunity to serve as Speaker of the House of Delegates of the American Dietetic Association in 1991.

Several awards have also come my way, including Recognized Young Dietitian of the Year from the Oklahoma Dietetic Association, HRSA Administrators Award for Excellence in Health Promotion from the Indian Health Service, the Secretary's Award for Exceptional Achievement from the United States Department of Health and Human Services, and an Award of Merit from the Oregon Dietetic Association.

While I stay busy with professional activities, I also make sure that I have time to enjoy my hobbies of reading English mysteries, walking, and watching for whales on the Pacific Coast. During my years in the Pacific Northwest, I have also developed an appreciation for the Northwest Indian arts and crafts.

My advice to aspiring dietetics professionals is to study hard, seize every opportunity to learn and have new experiences, and have fun in your profession. A sense of humor is invaluable, along with a genuine love of people. Keep these things in mind and you'll go far in your profession!

CHAPTER 4

$\blacklozenge$

The Dietary Managers Association

A brochure from the Dietary Managers Association states, "If you have enjoyed a hot lunch at school, been admitted to a hospital, or shared dinner with a family member or friend in a nursing home, chances are you had indirect contact with a professional dietary manager."[1] Who is the dietary manager?

The membership of the Dietary Managers Association (DMA), shows that dietetic management is a young profession on the move. Membership in the DMA has increased by more than 13,000 in just over 30 years.

Members of this association have been trained in foodservice operations management. In partnership with dietitians, they usually supervise and manager dietetic services in long-term care facilities, hospitals, schools, the military, correctional institutions, and other non-commercial foodservice operations.

The DMA promotes and maintains the competency of its members by making a certified credential available. The certified dietary manager must pass a competency exam and participate in a specified number of hours of continuing education. Like the ADA, the DMA has adopted a Code of Ethics to promote and maintain the highest standards of professional and personal conduct among its members. In addition, a wide array of benefits are available to members of the association.

FROM THE BEGINNING

In 1960, the Hospital, Institution, and Educational Food Service Society (HIEFSS) was founded and incorporated in the State of Illinois. The first meeting of HIEFSS was held in Cleveland, Ohio and was attended by 72 prospective members from 15 different states. Representatives from The American Dietetic Association were also present, and participated actively in all decisions made at this meeting. The Board of Directors of the new association was established with five voting members. The Board was expanded to 15 voting members in 1978, as part of a reorganization of the association.[2]

The most common title used by members in 1960 was *foodservice supervisor*. In an effort to develop a career ladder of titles within the dietetics profession, the leadership of The American Dietetic Association changed the title designation to *dietetic assistant* in 1971. A role-delineation study was conducted by Ohio State University between 1981 and 1983. This study was underwritten by HIEFSS and the Certifying Board for Dietary Managers. As a result, the designated professional title was changed to *dietary manager*.

In July 1984, HIEFSS became the Dietary Managers Association. Following the establishment of the certifying board for dietary managers, the first credentialing examination was offered in 1985. In 1984, DMA and Purdue University entered into an agreement which established the Center for Professional Development. In 1985, Purdue granted continuing education credits to those attending educational sessions at the DMA annual meeting. Under the auspices of the Center, Purdue faculty develop and present Skill Builder Workshops designed around the ten areas of responsibility identified by the role-delineation studies. A correspondence course on Professional Cooking was also developed and has been used by individuals in this country as well as in England, Australia, Italy, and Canada.

Membership in the Dietary Managers Association exceeded 14,000 in 1994; more than 9,000 of these members were certified.[3] Public relations activities, such as the dissemination of press releases, placement of commercial advertising, and promotions of free brochures are a major part of the Association's mission.

Although some facilities and educational programs continue to call trained individuals *foodservice supervisors*, the DMA works diligently to promote use of the title *dietary manager*. Currently, two-thirds of DMA members have been certified. One state requires that all dietary managers be certified; similar legislation is being considered by several other states.

To recognize the work of foodservice staff DMA established Pride in Food Service Week in 1991. Merchandise—such as posters, buttons, and tee shirts—is sold each year to promote this celebration and DMA brochures offer suggestions for other ways to celebrate.[4]

MEMBERSHIP CATEGORIES

The DMA has four categories of membership. Active membership in the association has always required the completion of a specific training program, including both classroom learning and supervised practice experience. **Active Membership** is available to those who have graduated from a dietary managers training program approved by DMA. **Active Certified Membership** is offered to those individuals who have completed the DMA-approved training program, passed the credentialing exam, and applied for certification.[5]

Individuals who have completed an associate, bachelor's, or advanced degree in foodservice, health care, or a related field may become **associate members**. All membership benefits are available to Associate Members, except the right to vote or hold office. **Student Membership** is open to those currently enrolled in a DMA-approved training program. Student members, too, are eligible for all benefits except voting privileges and holding office. Students are not eligible to take the credentialing exam until they have completed the training program.

THE CERTIFIED CREDENTIAL

C.D.M. (Certified Dietary Manager) may be listed after a dietary manager's name when he or she has passed a competency exam administered by a testing firm and applied for certification through the Certifying Board for Dietary Managers. The Certifying Board is independent of DMA and comprised of six individuals—three members of DMA, and three representatives of the allied professions, the general public, and employers of dietary managers.

Five categories of people are eligible to take the dietary managers credentialing exam: (1) Active members of DMA; (2) Nonmembers of DMA who have completed a DMA-approved dietary managers course; (3) Nonmembers of DMA who hold a two- or four-year degree in foodservice management and nutrition; (4) Associate members of DMA with a two- or four-year degree in foodservice management and nutrition; and (5) Associate members of DMA who have graduated from a state-approved or other accredited course and who have two years of experience (80% management/20% nutrition).

The certifying exam assesses competency in the areas of responsibility identified by the role-delineation studies. There are 175 multiple choice questions based on critical incident scenarios. The examinee must read a description of a situation and choose the appropriate response from the multiple choices offered. Three and a half hours are allowed for completion of the exam. The ten areas covered by the test and the percentage of questions from each area are shown in the following outline. The exam outline provides a thorough and accurate list of the responsibilities included in a dietary manager's job description.

1. Patient/Client Nutrition—Gather Nutrition Data: 11 percent
   a. Document and file nutritional information in medical records
   b. Interview patients/clients for diet history

   c. Conduct routine nutritional screening to identify non-problem cases

   d. Calculate nutrition intake, such as calories and sodium

   e. Identify nutrition problems and needs

2. Patient/Client Nutrition—Apply Nutrition Data: 6 percent

   a. Implement diet plans or menus using appropriate modifications

   b. Implement physician's routine dietary orders

   c. Utilize standard nutritional care procedures

   d. Conduct routine evaluation of effectiveness of nutritional care plan

3. Patient/Client Service—Provide Foodservice: 9 percent

   a. Check trayline for food quality, portion size, and diet accuracy

   b. Supervise the preparation and serving of special nourishment and supplemental feedings

   c. Develop foodservice quality control procedures

   d. Evaluate food acceptance survey and plate waste data

   e. Identify appropriate resources to modify standard menus to suit patient's needs

4. Patient/Client—Provide Nutrition Education: 8 percent

   a. Help patients/clients choose foods from selective menus

   b. Select and use nutrition education materials

   c. Teach patients/clients how to plan and prepare prescribed meals

5. Food Facility Personnel—Hire and Supervise: 13 percent

   a. Develop and maintain employee schedules

   b. Prepare daily work assignment

   c. Conduct employee performance evaluation

   d. Interview and select employees

   e. Supervise, discipline, and recommend promotion/termination

6. Food Facility Personnel—Develop Personnel Communications: 5 percent

   a. Implement required changes in food facility

   b. Prepare, plan, and conduct facility meetings

   c. Present work procedures and plans

   d. Teach employees

   e. Recommend improvements in facility design and layout

   f. Set goals and priorities for facility

7. Food Facility Personnel—Develop External Relations: 10 percent

   a. Represent facility at external meetings

   b. Coordinate facility services and plans with outside groups

   c. Communicate patient/client information to other health professionals

   d. Participate in patient/client care conferences and case presentations

   e. Participate in a medical audit of patient/client care

8. Food/Kitchen—Manage Supplies, Equipment Use, Sanitation and Safety: 18 percent

   a. Receive, store, and distribute food supplies and equipment

   b. Prepare and maintain inventory records

   c. Follow standard sanitation and infectious disease control practices

   d. Write cleaning procedures for utensils, equipment, and work areas

   e. Conduct routine safety inspection of work areas

   f. Conduct routine maintenance inspection of equipment

   g. Instruct employees in equipment use and maintenance

   h. Organize work-flow and use of equipment

   i. Write procedures to comply with health-care standards

9. Food/Kitchen—Manage Production and Facilities: 13 percent

    a. Prepare standard recipes for food production

    b. Specify standards and procedures for preparing food

    c. Identify equipment needs

    d. Test new recipes

    e. Supervise the production and distribution of food

10. Financial—Manage Business Operations: 7 percent

    a. Write purchase specifications and orders

    b. Supervise cafeteria cash activities and reports

    c. Calculate cost and set prices for catered events

    d. Write detailed specifications for major appliances needed

    e. Evaluate price bids and decide on vendors

    f. Supervise the purchase of food and supplies

    g. Recommend salary and wage adjustments for employees

    h. Monitor/review cost of menus against budget and guidelines[6]

Passing the exam certifies that the individual is capable of competently performing the entry-level responsibilities expected of a professional dietary manager.

In order to maintain the CDM credential, an individual must earn 45 hours of continuing education credit every three years. This requirement ensures that the certified dietary manager remains up-to-date on the latest information in the field of dietary management.

THE DMA CODE OF ETHICS

One of the requirements of a profession is that it regulate the ethical conduct of its members. DMA promotes and maintaining the highest standards of professional and personal conduct among its members through the adoption and enforcement of its code of ethics. Adherence to the code is required for membership.

Code of Ethics

As a member of Dietary Managers Association, I pledge myself to:

- Reflect my pride in my competence as a dietary manager by wearing my pin and emblem and displaying my certificate.
- Use only legal and ethical means in the practice of my profession.
- Use every opportunity to improve public understanding of the role of the dietary manager.
- Promote and encourage the highest level of ethics within the industry.
- Refuse to engage in, or countenance, activities for personal gain at the expense of my employer, the industry, or the profession.
- Maintain the confidentiality of privileged information entrusted or known to me by virtue of my position.
- Maintain loyalty to my employers, and pursue their objectives in ways that are consistent with the public interest.
- Always communicate the administrative decisions of my employer in a truthful and accurate manner.
- Communicate to proper authorities, but disclose to no one else, any evidence of infraction of established rules and regulations.
- Strive for excellence in all aspects of management and nutritional practices, with constant attention to self-improvement.
- Maintain the highest standard of personal conduct.[7]

BENEFITS OF MEMBERSHIP IN DMA

The major emphasis of DMA is education and continuing education. An annual meeting is held which includes exhibits and educational programs. District, state, and national meetings feature speakers on topics of relevance to the field. The Center for Professional Development makes educational programs available across the country.

The Dietary Manager magazine is published bimonthly and sent to all members. It includes nutrition and management feature articles, product information, legislative news, book reviews, classified advertising, tips for professional development, and professional association information. Several reference books are produced by DMA and offered to members at reduced prices.

DMA is headquartered in Illinois; it has a Washington, D.C. office to monitor and impact legislation affecting dietary managers. At the grassroots level, volunteer efforts like letter-writing campaigns are used to influence pending health-care reform legislation.

Participation on a local level offers members education, camaraderie, peer support, and opportunities for networking. Holding an office in DMA offers personal and professional gratification and the opportunity to further develop leadership abilities.

The DMA employment exchange program is available free to members and confidentially matches job seekers with a computer-generated listing of job openings in the desired locale. This computer database is maintained by the membership services department and may be used by job seekers and those who have employment opportunities.

DMA encourages members to call its toll-free number [(800)603–5838] for answers to their questions regarding current trends, education opportunities, association activities, and any other areas of need. Members receive a certificate of membership suitable for framing and a plastic membership card. Optional benefits include group-rate insurance programs, a VISA card with the association's logo on it, and special car rental rates.

SUMMARY

DMA's slogan says it all: "The Dietary Managers Association is an organization of professionals dedicated to achieving excellence in the food service industry." This relatively young professional association sets high ideals for itself and its members. Standards of professional and personal conduct have been carefully written and communicated to the membership. The standards are measurable and attainable and serve to define the profession.

Membership is limited to those who have met the requisite educational standards, which include both academic learning and hands-on experience in approved programs. Those who aspire to an advanced level of professional status may demonstrate their competence by successfully completing a credentialing exam.

The primary focus of DMA is educational. Opportunities are provided for member education via publications, meetings, exhibits, a bimonthly magazine, workshops, and courses. DMA also provides members with peer support, professional recognition, public relations for the profession, opportunities for networking, career guidance, legislative representation, and other valuable benefits.

SUGGESTED ACTIVITIES

1. Locate a dietary manager in your area and interview him or her. A local community college or technical school that offers the DMA-approved training course would be a good resource.

2. Compare and contrast the certified dietary manager credential to that of the registered dietitian. How are they alike and how do they differ?

3. A strong working relationship exists between the dietitian and the dietary manager. Describe why this is the case and how this relationship manifests itself.

NOTES

1. Dietary Managers Association. *Answers to your questions about dietary managers.*

2. Dietary Managers Association. *History of Dietary Managers Association.* Dietary Managers Association; 1985.

3. St. John W. A look at the year ahead for DMA. *Dietary Manager,* 1994;3:32.

4. Dietary Managers Association. Tips for celebrating Pride in Food Service Week. *Dietary Manager,* 1993;2:27–29.

5. Dietary Managers Association. *Invest in your professional success with Dietary Managers Association.*

6. Dietary Managers Association. *CBDM Credentialing Exam.*

7. Dietary Managers Association, *Code of Ethics.*

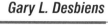

Gary L. Desbiens

Parkview Memorial Hospital
Wiscasset, Maine

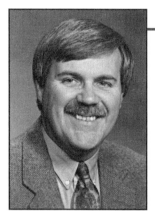

When I decided to return to college at the age of 31, I had no idea what a rewarding career I had chosen. I enrolled in a two-year ADA-approved program in dietetic technology at the local community college. In 1983, I graduated with an associate degree and accepted a position as a clinical dietetic technician at a large, inner-city teaching hospital.

In 1984, I became involved in professional organizations and was elected president-elect and then president of the Connecticut Dietetic Technician Special Interest Group. This involvement proved to be a very valuable experience for me, teaching me leadership skills and challenging me to become active in the state dietetic association. I was selected the Recognized Dietetic Technician of the year for Connecticut, and this award opened doors for me to become involved on a national level. In 1986, I was asked by The American Dietetic Association to serve on the House of Delegates Committee on Association Membership.

In 1984, I decided to continue my education and enrolled in a general dietetics program at the University of New Haven. Following the completion of a bachelor's degree in 1989, I moved to Maine where I was employed as an assistant director of nutrition services in a small community hospital. Two years later I became director.

As director of nutrition services I am responsible for overseeing the preparation and delivery of 7,000 meals per month in three divisions—patient tray line, cafeteria, and catering. My facility, which is run by Seventh Day Adventists, is somewhat unique in that all the meals served in the cafeteria and catered events are strictly vegetarian. The challenge of my position lies in planning meals that are not only vegetarian, but are also low-fat, healthy, and good-tasting.

A career in dietetics has been rewarding for me. What I like most about the field is the diversity and versatility. The availability of networking opportunities is another favorable aspect of dietetics. I think most dietetics professionals would agree that the thing they like least is keeping up with changes. The current need to do more with less—which is prevalent everywhere—is a constant challenge.

My advice to future practitioners is to seek challenge and to gain a wide variety of experiences in as many practice settings as possible. The times are rapidly changing. Practitioners may be finding themselves responsible for areas never before explored and thus need to be multiskilled. Development of management skills is essential and continual learning is critical. Future practitioners should be focused on their goals and keep in mind that they alone hold the key to success in a rewarding career.

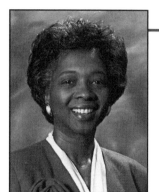

Yvonne Lafayette Cade Bronner

*The Johns Hopkins University
Baltimore, Maryland*

I grew up in a small town of Elberton, Georgia, and I had never heard the word *dietitian* until I was in college. I was first interested in fashion design and was majoring in home economics when I first learned about dietetics. I was attracted to the field because it is linked to service and interaction with people, while it allows for creative expression through the art and science of food. After graduating, I did not do an internship but worked for brief periods in hospital and community dietetics while being a homemaker. It was while studying for my master of science degree in public health nutrition at Case Western Reserve University that I became excited about working in the community and a career as a public health nutritionist. Following graduation, I taught at Cuyahoga Community College in Cleveland, and later was an instructor at Westchester Community College in Valhalla, New York. I became a registered dietitian in 1974.

My work with public health in the Maternal and Infant Program and later with the WIC Program was very enjoyable and solidified my interest in public health nutrition. This interest and experience led me to pursue doctoral studies, earning a doctor of science degree from Johns Hopkins University in 1983. I immediately joined the faculty at Howard University in Washington, D.C., where I conducted research in the area of breast-feeding promotion and peer counseling. It was also during this time that I was appointed to the ADA Ambassador

Program and became a media spokesperson for that organization.

My current position is at Johns Hopkins University in the Department of Maternal and Child Health. My responsibilities include teaching, research, student advisement, and community service. My research focuses on breast-feeding promotion among urban African-American women and nutrition education/behavior change. One very rewarding breast-feeding promotion for me was serving as principal investigator for the grant that developed *Giving You the Best That I Got, Baby*, a breast-feeding promotional video with singer Anita Baker.

Participation in the ADA Ambassador Program opened a window of opportunity and vision for me. As a result of the extensive media training and practice with radio, TV, and print media, I learned that I enjoyed interacting with the public at this level and became much more involved in public speaking. The vision of improved nutrition through communication is exciting and continues to be very rewarding.

Dietetics is a great profession because of the breadth of career choices. The sky and your imagination set the limits. One of my greatest concerns is the low number of students and dietitians from minority groups. This is especially troubling since much of the work in public health involves service to these populations.

Good nutrition and moderate exercise are the two major modifiable behavioral health factors that can improve the health of the nation. Whether your career choice is clinical dietetics, public health, education, research, or foodservice, you can make a measurable difference in the future health of the nation by communicating nutrition messages effectively.

CHAPTER 5

$\diamond$

Dietetic Education and Training

O ne of the first actions of the fledgling ADA was the establishment of a teaching section, to provide guidance in the education and training of dietitians.[1] Through the years, the ADA has continued to be mindful of the education of future professionals, modifying educational standards to meet the ever-changing needs of the marketplace.

Two major study commissions, one in 1972 and another in 1984, were formed to make recommendations regarding the many questions facing dietetic education.[2] Other task forces, such as the Task Force on Education in 1982, the Critical Issues Task Force in 1992, and the Dietetic Education Task Force in 1993, have also addressed issues of importance to the educational process.[3]

What knowledge, skills, and abilities are necessary for successful dietetics practice? Should there be dietetic specialties? What kind of preparation is necessary for specialization? Should dietetic education programs be approved or accredited? How are entry-level practice and advanced practice different? The questions could go on and on: dietetic education programs are always evolving as the profession of dietetics continues to change and grow.

A BRIEF HISTORY OF DIETETIC EDUCATION REQUIREMENTS

In 1923, dietetic educators first outlined the courses they believed were necessary to prepare a student for dietetics practice. In 1927, the "Outline for Standard Course for Student Dietitians in Hospitals" was approved by the ADA. This document required that students have a baccalaureate degree with a major in foods and nutrition and at least six months of training in a hospital (Figure 5.1) under the direction of a dietitian. The first list of hospitals offering this approved course was published in 1928.

In 1947, the academic expectations for students entering internships were published and became known as Plan I. Plan II, which covered four subject areas with a range of semester hours was introduced in 1955. Plan III, begun in 1958, approached the educational process by designating core subjects, emphases, and concentrations. Plan IV, which included competency-based minimum academic requirements, was published in 1971. In 1987, Plan V was implemented, with *Knowledge Requirements for Dietitians*

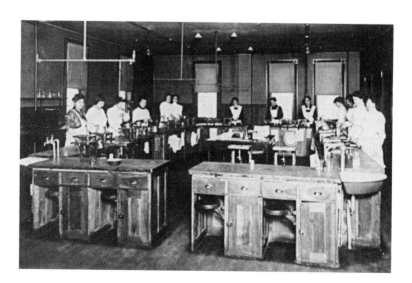

Figure 5.1
A very early food science laboratory.
Photo courtesy of The American Dietetic Association.

(Figure 5.2). Plan V also specified *Performance Requirements for Entry-Level Dietitians* (see Figure 5.3) to describe the skills which must be demonstrated or performed by those completing the supervised practice component of a dietetic education program. In 1987, the Council on Education of the ADA voted to discontinue the numbering of its educational plans. The *Standards of Education* were introduced as the minimum criteria to be met by all dietetic education programs.

For many years, the only way to become a dietitian was to complete a post-baccalaureate dietetic internship. However, in 1962 the first Coordinated Undergraduate Program in Dietetics was developed. This type of program combined the required internship with the academic program. The student's hands-on experiences were coordinated with what was being discussed in the classroom, with the goal of making this combined learning experience even more meaningful. Through the Coordinated Undergraduate Program a student could fulfill the academic and experience requirements in four years rather than five.

In the early 1970s, the need for dietetic support personnel led to the development of associate degree programs for dietetic technicians. These programs combined a two-year associate degree with 450 hours of hands-on experience. In 1974, guidelines for approving dietetic technician programs were introduced.

In the 1980s, Approved Pre-Professional Practice Programs, known as AP4s, were developed. These post-baccalaureate programs were similar to dietetic internships, but provided some new features. AP4s were introduced as a means of encouraging the sponsorship of dietetic education programs by nontraditional dietetic practice settings such as business and industry, public health departments, or school districts. The AP4s enabled students to complete program requirements through part-time work.

In 1993, the Dietetic Education Task Force recommended that all post-baccalaureate supervised practice programs would become known as *internships* and

1. Knows principles of effective oral and written communication and documentation.
2. Knows fundamentals of human relations and group dynamics.
3. Knows techniques of interviewing and counseling.
4. Knows principles of education and effective methods of teaching.
5. Knows use of computers for data processing and information management in dietetics.
6. Knows basic concepts of research methodology and statistical analysis.
7. Knows fundamentals of quality assurance.
8. Knows laws, regulations, and standards affecting dietetic practice.
9. Knows principles of human anatomy and physiology, microbiology, organic chemistry, and biochemistry.
10. Knows principles of behavioral and social sciences.
11. Knows the physiological, biochemical, and behavioral bases for nutrition intervention in health and disease.
12. Knows the influence of socioeconomic, cultural, and psychological factors on food and nutrition behavior.
13. Knows energy and nutrient needs for various stages of the life cycle.
14. Knows principles of food science and techniques of food preparation.
15. Knows nutrient composition of food and appropriate sources of data.
16. Knows principles of menu planning for optimal nutrition of individuals and groups in health and disease.
17. Knows principles of nutrition screening, assessment, planning, intervention, evaluation, and documentation.
18. Knows resources for delivery of nutrition care in community programs.
19. Knows principles of procurement, food production, distribution, and service.
20. Knows fundamentals and techniques of financial management.
21. Knows principles of organization and management.
22. Knows principles and techniques of human resource management.
23. Knows fundamentals of marketing food and nutrition services.
24. Knows fundamentals of the political and legislative process.

Figure 5.2

Knowledge Requirements for Entry-Level Dietitians
Accreditation/Approval Manual for Dietetic Education Programs.
2nd ed. Chicago: The American Dietetic Association; 1991.

1. Utilizes effective oral and written communication skills in the practice of dietetics.
2. Promotes effective professional relationships in the practice of dietetics.
3. Provides education to consumers, clients, other professionals, and support personnel.
4. Utilizes computer and other technologies in the practice of dietetics.
5. Applies current research information in the practice of dietetics.
6. Participates in quality assurance programs.
7. Utilizes knowledge of political, legislative, and economic factors that affect dietetic practice.
8. Complies with the Code of Ethics and Standards of Practice for the Profession of Dietetics.
9. Provides nutrition care for individuals and groups through systematic screening, assessment, planning, intervention, evaluation, and documentation.
10. Provides nutrition counseling and education to individuals and groups for health promotion, maintenance, treatment, and rehabilitation.
11. Participates in the management of cost-effective nutrition care systems.
12. Utilizes food, nutrition, and social service resources in community programs.
13. Assures that foodservice operations meet the food and nutrition needs of target markets.
14. Utilizes menus as focal points for control of the foodservice system.
15. Participates in the management of foodservice systems, including procurement, food production, distribution, and service.
16. Participates in the management of human, financial, material, physical, and operational resources.
17. Integrates food and nutrition services with other services in the practice setting.
18. Participates in activities that promote improved nutrition status of consumers and market the profession of dietetics.

Figure 5.3
Performance Requirements for Entry-Level Dietitians
Accreditation/Approval Manual for Dietetic Education Programs.
2nd ed. Chicago: The American Dietetic Association; 1991.

their participants as *interns*. Thus, the distinction between AP4s and dietetic internships will be eliminated in the years ahead, reducing the confusion which surrounds the two types of post-baccalaureate supervised practice programs.

ADA'S STANDARDS OF EDUCATION AND THE ACCREDITATION/APPROVAL PROCESS

The ADA's Standards of Education outline five prerequisites that must be met by every dietetic education program:

1. The philosophy and goals of the program shall provide guidance to the program.
2. The accountability of a program to its students shall be identified.
3. Resources available to the program shall be identified and their contribution to the program described.
4. The curriculum shall provide for development of expected competence of the program graduate.
5. A systematic approach shall be used in managing and evaluating the program.

Before a dietetic program can begin accepting students, the program's director and faculty members must undertake an in-depth review process known as a *self-study*. The process for conducting a self-study is outlined in ADA's *Accreditation/Approval Manual for Dietetic Education Programs*.[4] The self-study document outlines in detail how the dietetic program meets the ADA Standards of Education. The written self-study document is then forwarded to a review panel of the Commission on Accreditation/Approval for Dietetics Education (CAADE).

A dietetic education program which offers only the coursework necessary to meet the *Knowledge Requirements for the Entry-Level Dietitian* is called a *Didac-*

tic Program in Dietetics (DPD). If this program submits a self-study which acceptably demonstrates how it meets the five Standards of Education, the program becomes an *approved* dietetic education program, meaning that it passed a pencil-and-paper review by the CAADE. A site visit, where representatives of the CAADE actually visit the dietetics program, is not conducted for DPDs.

Since Coordinated Programs in Dietetics provide both the academic component and the supervised practice component, the self-study for a CP must outline how it meets both the *Knowledge Requirements* and the *Performance Requirements for Entry-Level Dietitians.* Once the pencil-and-paper review of the self-study document is completed by the CAADE Review Panel, two or three site visitors are dispatched to visit the program and verify that what was presented in the self-study document is actually occurring. The site visit is a required step for coordinated programs and dietetic memberships seeking to be accredited by the CAADE. The pencil-and-paper review and the site visit assure students, parents, administrators, and others that the dietetic education program meets the high standards set by the American Dietetic Association.

THE THREE STEPS TO BECOMING A REGISTERED DIETITIAN (R.D.) OR DIETETIC TECHNICIAN, REGISTERED (D.T.R.)

There are three components in the preparation for dietetics practice: education, supervised practice, and credentialing. These three steps apply whether you wish to become a dietetic technician, registered (DTR) or a registered dietitian (RD).

To become a D.T.R., you must:

1. Complete a two-year associate degree in an accredited dietetic technician program which meets the *Knowledge Requirements for Dietetic Technicians* outlined by the ADA Council on Education.

2. Complete a minimum of 450 hours of supervised practice experience that meets the *Performance Requirements for Dietetic Technicians.* This experience must be gained under the direction of an accredited dietetic technician program.

3. Successfully complete the national Registration Examination for Dietetic Technicians.

To become an R.D., you must:

1. Complete a baccalaureate degree in an approved didactic program in dietetics or an accredited coordinated program in dietetics that meets the *Knowledge Requirements for Entry-Level Dietitians* outlined by the ADA Council on Education.

2. Complete a minimum of 900 hours of supervised practice experience within an accredited coordinated program, an accredited dietetic internship, or an approved pre-professional practice program that meets the *Performance Requirements for Entry-Level Dietitians.*

3. Successfully complete the national Registration Examination for Dietitians.

The Academic Experience

The academic preparation to become a dietitian may be obtained in either an approved didactic program or an accredited coordinated program in dietetics. The dietetics curriculum may be slightly different at different universities, because each school has unique strengths and resources. Graduates of DPDs are eligible to apply for post-baccalaureate supervised practice programs in order to meet ADA's requirements. Graduates of a coordinated program in dietetics meet both academic and supervised practice requirements in their degree program.

A typical dietetics curriculum might include courses such as written communications, speech, psychology, sociology, economics, and humanities courses. Courses in biology, anatomy and physiology, microbiology, chemistry, organic chemistry, and biochemistry are also required. Support courses often include organization and management, accounting, marketing, educational theory, or other courses. Professional courses might include normal nutrition, clinical nutrition, public health nutrition, food science, quantity food production, and foodservice purchasing. Students who are participating in a coordinated program in dietetics will have courses that have a supervised practice component.

The *Directory of Dietetics Programs 1994–1995*[5] lists 233 didactic programs approved by the American Dietetic Association. There are didactic programs in dietetics in the District of Columbia, Puerto Rico, and all states except Alaska. Some states have numerous programs: Texas has 17 programs and California and Illinois each have 15 approved programs. There are currently 51 coordinated programs in dietetics accredited by the American Dietetic Association, in 28 states.

Students seeking admission to supervised practice programs should realize that grade point average, particularly in the physical and biological sciences, is an important criteria for acceptance. Many supervised practice programs look for applicants with at least a 3.0 grade point average (on a 4.0 scale) to be considered for appointment. A solid academic base is essential for success in a supervised practice experience.

The Supervised Practice Experience

The American Dietetic Association requires a minimum of 900 hours of supervised practice experience, which may be obtained in a coordinated program, dietetic internship, or pre-professional practice program. Dietetic internships and pre-professional practice programs are post-baccalaureate experiences for graduates of didactic programs. Supervised practice experience has already been completed by graduates of a coordinated program.

Supervised practice experience in a pre-professional practice program or dietetic internship may be either full-time (40 hours per week) or part-time (20 hours per week). However, the program must be specifically designed with a part-time component for the student to utilize this approach. Supervised practice in a coordinated program in dietetics may vary from a few hours per week at the junior level to 30–35 hours per week at the senior level. Most supervised practice experiences are unpaid, although some post-baccalaureate experiences do provide a stipend. The *Directory of Dietetics Programs 1994–1995* provides information on stipends, length of programs, number of students accepted per class, and other important information.

Some post-baccalaureate supervised practice programs combine the opportunity to earn graduate credits or even a complete master's degree with the supervised practice experience. Some programs *require* a master's degree in conjunction with the practical experience; other programs make completion of the graduate degree optional. Students applying for these programs must meet the graduate-school requirements of the institution to which they are applying. Typically, a minimum grade point average of 3.0 is required. Many programs also require that the applicant submit scores from the Graduate Records Examination (GRE) as part of the supervised practice program application. Applicants should contact the program director to obtain information on a specific supervised practice program.

Students applying for pre-professional practice programs or dietetic internships must participate in a computer matching process. The computer matching program compares each applicant's rank-ordered list of programs she/he is interested in with supervised practice programs' rank-ordered list of individuals they would like to see in their program. When a match is found, the student is notified for acceptance or rejection of the placement. Students may apply to as many programs as they wish, but the computer match forces students to rank their list and make some decisions about which program seems best to them.

Supervised practice experiences are based on the *Performance Requirements for Entry-Level Dietitians.* Supervised practice programs, like their didactic counterparts, are designed to take advantage of the strengths and expertise of each program's faculty and staff. All supervised practice programs provide experiences in nutrition services delivery, community nutrition or public health nutrition, and foodservice systems management, although the amount of time spent in each of these areas varies from program to program. ADA does not mandate equal emphasis in the three areas, but does expect that all areas will be covered in the supervised practice program.

The supervised practice experience is one of the most meaningful parts of preparation for dietetics practice. The opportunity to work alongside practicing dietetic professionals is exciting and challenging and the hands-on experiences bring the information presented during the academic program to life. Thus, the supervised practice experience is an important step in helping students move from theory to the reality of dietetic practice.

Supervised practice experiences are designed to move from simple to complex, from functioning with assistance to functioning alone, from student to entry-level dietitian. Frequently, a student will observe a task being performed by a dietitian or dietetic technician. Next, the student will attempt the activity with guidance from the professional. Finally, the student progresses to independent functioning. At each step, students are evaluated and specific feedback is provided to enhance the learning experience. Early experiences may involve role-playing or other forms of simulation so that students can develop skills in a low-risk environment. As skill levels and confidence increase, the student is allowed to take on more and more responsibility. Culminating experiences, such as "staff relief," allow the student to function independently as a full-fledged dietitian and, thus, give the student a realistic picture of dietetics practice.

Verification of Education and Supervised Practice Experience

Upon successful completion of the education and supervised practice components, the student is issued a verification statement. This form is a legal document and should be treated as such. This document, bearing the original signature of the program director, verifies that the student successfully completed the education and/or supervised practice experience. Students completing a DPD and a post-baccalaureate supervised practice program will have two verification statements; students completing a coordinated program will have only one form. These statements must be presented when the student changes from associate to active membership in the ADA. Likewise, these statements must be included in the application packet for the national Registration Examination for Dietitians.

Students enrolled in a dietetic technician program must also present a verification statement before sitting for the national Registration Examination for Dietetic Technicians. Since dietetic technician programs combine education with supervised practice, only one verification statement is issued upon program completion.

SUMMARY

Preparation for entry into the profession of dietetics encompasses both prescribed academic preparation and supervised hands-on experience. Both of these components are carefully structured and monitored by the ADA through its Council on Professional Issues and the Commission on Accreditation/Approval for Dietetics Education. On-going role delineation studies form the basis for the *Knowledge and Performance*

Statements used to guide the development of both academic curricula and supervised practice experiences.

The challenge facing ADA and dietetic educators is to keep educational preparation on the cutting edge of professional practice, ensuring that current students will be prepared for the exciting future that awaits them as dietetic technicians and registered dietitians. The most important focus must be on the development of critical thinking and problem-solving skills, so that future dietitians know HOW to think, rather than WHAT to think. You must be prepared to take responsibility for your own continued professional development, since information about food and nutrition issues is expanding at an exponential rate. Learn how to learn, and you will be ready for an exciting future in dietetics.

SUGGESTED ACTIVITIES

1. Find out about the history of your dietetics program. When did the program begin? How many people have graduated from your program? What are some of those graduates doing now?

2. Interview a dietitian in your area. Find out the following information:

   a. How did you learn about the profession of dietetics?

   b. What kind of dietetics education program did you go through?

   c. What was your first dietetics position?

   d. What other dietetics positions have you held?

   e. Describe your current job and its responsibilities.

   f. What skills do you believe are necessary for successful dietetics practice?

   g. What do you like best about being a dietitian or dietetic technician?

3. Obtain a copy of the *Directory of Dietetics Programs* from your program director. Are there other dietetics education programs in your state? in a neighboring state? If so, where are they? What kinds of programs are offered? Contact some of the students in these programs and network with them!

NOTES

1. Cassell J. *Carry the Flame: The History of the American Dietetic Association.* Chicago: The American Dietetic Association; 1990.

2. *The Profession of Dietetics. The Report of the Study Commission on Dietetics.* Chicago: The American Dietetic Association; 1972. *A New Look at the Profession of Dietetics: Report of the 1984 Study Commission on Dietetics.* Chicago: The American Dietetic Association; 1984.

3. Haschke MB, Maize RS. President's Page: Dietetic education: The future and policy decisions. *Journal of the American Dietetic Association,* 1984;84:208–212. *Report of the Critical Issues: Registration Eligibility and Licensure Task Force.* The American Dietetic Association; 1992 (unpublished). *Report of the Dietetic Education Task Force.* The American Dietetic Association; 1993 (unpublished).

4. *Accreditation/Approval Manual for Dietetic Education Programs.* Chicago: The American Dietetic Association.

5. *Directory of Dietetics Programs 1994–1995.* Chicago: The American Dietetic Association; 1994.

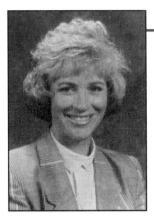

Cathy Miller

*National Steak and Poultry
City of Industry, California*

M y interest in dietetics dates back to high school. At a College Night as a junior in high school, my mother handed me a brochure on career opportunities with a degree in food science and nutrition, and I was hooked. I chose to attend Colorado State University. Once there, I learned about becoming a registered dietitian, and became determined to attain that credential. I also took the advice of one of my professors and sought various kinds of work experience while in college. I worked in a donut shop and in the kitchen of a local hospital, volunteered for the city's soup kitchen by planning menus and serving food, and taught basic cooking classes at a local home for unwed mothers. Looking back, the experience I am most thankful for was a 12-hour per week "internship" I had one summer in test kitchens for Current, Inc. To support myself during the internship, I worked in the pantry and bakery of a nearby country club.

I completed my dietetic internship at the University of California Medical Center in San Francisco. After interning, I worked as a consultant for Beatrice/Hunt–Wesson, testing and developing recipes and determining label directions for both retail and foodservice products. Six months after passing the RD exam, I began an intermediate culinary course at the Cordon Blue School of Cookery in London, England. The program taught me such things as presentation, proper seasoning of dishes, and food preparation from scratch, all with the freshest of ingredients but without the use of power-driven devices. Cooking school filled in gaps in my formal dietetics education.

After traveling a bit in Europe, I spent two years in Menomonie, Wisconsin, earning a master's degree in food science and nutrition, focusing mostly on food and foodservice. Upon graduation, I began working in Research and Development for Foodmaker, Inc., developing and implementing new menu items for Jack in the Box restaurants. After five years, I became director of the department, with a staff of ten and an annual budget of $875,000. I was the first dietitian hired by the company. Part of my responsibilities included updating the company's nutrition brochure every six months, handling customer affairs related to nutrition or new products, exhibiting at shows and events, and handling any ingredient formulation for improved nutrition profiles for our products.

My current position is director of research and development with National Steak and Poultry, a company which processes beef, poultry, and pork. We specialize in sizing, marinating, and freezing meat products for chain restaurants. My key responsibility is to ensure development of new products for existing or potential customers. Knowledge of food science, culinary principles, nutrition, computers, and foodservice operations is required. Communication skills are imperative. We use creativity in brainstorming new products, developing new flavor combinations, determining how to effectively produce a new item, and showing new menu presentations to customers.

Based on my experience, here are three tips for students planning a career in dietetics:

a. Get work experience, either paid or volunteer, while in school. This gives you a chance to find out if you are going to enjoy your career in this field and begin building your network of contacts.

b. Get involved in professional organizations now. By volunteering, you will be able to attend meetings, learn about job openings, and be in a prime networking position. Get your name out among these professionals.

c. Continue to pursue education in an area of interest outside of dietetics such as journalism, Spanish, computer science, business classes, public speaking, etc. The more you have to offer, the more doors that will be open to you. If you want to work in a nontraditional setting in dietetics, you will *need* expertise in other areas. Having this additional education will set you apart from other applicants for a job.

CHAPTER 6

◆

Dietetics Credentialing

Defining the competence required of practitioners is an important quality-assurance activity for any profession. According to Webster's, the word *credential* means "a letter or certificate given to a person to show that he has a right to confidence or to the exercise of a certain position or authority; that which gives credit; that which entitles to credit, confidence, etc., establishing reliability."[1] This is an appropriate description of the work of the Commission on Dietetic Registration (CDR).

THE COMMISSION ON DIETETIC REGISTRATION (CDR)

CDR, the credentialing arm of the ADA, was first called the Committee on Professional Registration. In 1969, it was charged with the implementation of dietetic registration. In November, 1975, CDR was made an independent unit of the ADA. CDR is responsible for all aspects of the registration process: standard-setting for registration eligibility, examination development and administration, credentialing, and recertification. CDR grants recognition of entry-level competence to dietitians who meet its standards and qualifications. These dietitians may use the legally protected professional designation *Registered Dietitian* or the initials *R.D.* Dietetic technicians who meet the standards and qualifications for technicians may use the legally protected professional designation *Dietetic Technician, Registered* or the initials D.T.R.

CDR was originally made up of eight persons elected by the ADA membership. In 1979, a public member, who represents users of the services of R.D.s and D.T.R.s, was added to the Commission. In 1990, a DTR representative became a member of CDR, to represent the interests of dietetic technicians. In 1994, a C.D.R.-certified specialist was appointed to the Commission. In 1995, a Fellow of the ADA representative was added to the Commission. In all, the Commission on Dietetic Registration comprises 12 members.

Dietetic Registration

The purpose of registration is to protect the nutritional health, safety, and welfare of the public by encouraging high standards of performance of persons practicing in the profession of dietetics.[2] Registration of dietitians began in 1969, providing a legally protected title for credentialed practitioners.[3] At its inception, registration required membership in the ADA, completion of an examination, and a continuing education requirement. More than 19,000 members of the ADA became registered during the initial enrollment period, when the examination was waived.[4] Currently, there are 55,531 R.D.s.[5] Membership in the ADA is no longer a requirement for R.D. status.

The role of the dietetic technician is not to be overlooked. Dietetic technicians were first admitted to membership in the ADA in 1975. Certification for Dietetic Technicians Registered (D.T.R.) became a reality in 1983. CDR currently recognizes 4,297 D.T.R.s.[6]

The Registration Examination

The development of the examinations for R.D. and D.T.R. status is rigorous. Figure 6.1 outlines the steps in CDR's test development program. **Role delineation** is the important first step in this process. A role delineation study is an in-depth research study with the goal of describing the knowledge and skills necessary to competently practice dietetics at a specified level (in this instance, entry level). Because the role delineation study surveys current practitioners in the field, using it as a basis for test development ensures that the certification test is job-related, representative of current practice, and geared to the appropriate level of responsibility.

From the role delineation study, a blueprint for building the examination must be developed. **Test specifications** include a description of what is to be tested, the proportion of the test to be devoted to various content areas, and the characteristics of acceptable test items. Because the test specifications come from the role delineation study, the test is valid and credible.

Test item development is an exciting but time-consuming experience. Test questions are developed by individuals trained in the specifics of test construction. Care is taken in choosing individuals who represent a diversity of practice, geographic, and ethnic backgrounds. Four criteria are applied to each test question: (1) the question must be relevant and critical to entry-level practice; (2) the question must be accurate, current, and clear; (3) the question must not reflect regional or institutional differences; and, (4) the question must conform to test specifications. Test items are reviewed by professional test editors and item writers before being pretested as unscored items on actual administered examinations.

During the **test assembly and review** process, a draft test is assembled from items in the computerized test bank. Experienced test reviewers appointed by CDR review the items for content accuracy, currency, and relevance to entry-level practice. They must also be sure that each item has one best answer. The assembled test undergoes final review by the CDR Examination Panel.

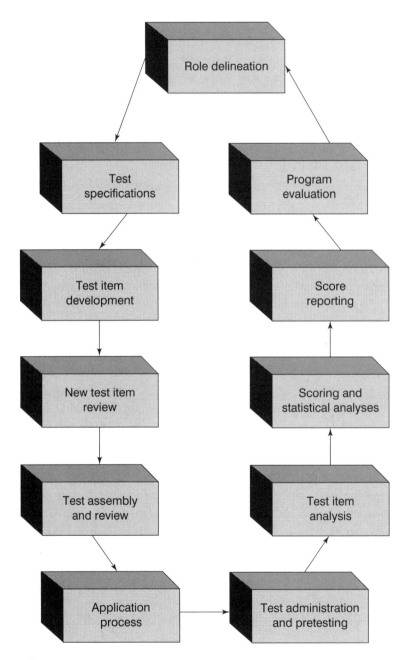

Figure 6.1
Certification Testing Program.
Reprinted with permission, Commission on Dietetic Registration.
The American Dietetic Association, Chicago, IL.

The R.D. and D.T.R. exams are held twice each year, in April and October. CDR works with the American College Testing Program (ACT) to administer the test at more than 80 sites nationwide. CDR will make special arrangements for such reasons as religious observance or physical handicap by arranging alternate test times or administration methods under secure standardized conditions.

After each test has been administered and items have been scored, psychometricians perform **test item analysis**. Performance statistics are reviewed for each test question in order to identify any problems. Test items that appear to be problematic are reviewed by experienced item-writers prior to score reporting, to eliminate any questions with ambiguities or response errors.

A **passing-score determination study** is periodically conducted by CDR, using experienced dietetics professionals from diverse practice areas and population subgroups. This passing score becomes the basis for evaluating future examinations, to ensure that all versions of the test are of equal difficulty.

Score reporting is two-fold. One report goes to the individual who took the examination. This report gives the test a total scaled score as well as raw scores in the different test domains or areas. CDR also provides, to dietetic education programs, both summary reports of the institution's graduates and individual scores if an examinee has authorized CDR to do so.[7]

Individuals who have completed both the academic preparation and supervised practice requirements and have received signed verification statements for both of these experiences may sit for the national Registration Examination for Dietitians or the Registration Examination for Dietetic Technicians. If an individual's degree was completed five or more years prior to applying to take the examination, six semester- or nine quarter-hours of dietetics-related coursework are required to update knowledge. Courses taken to satisfy the requirements must be completed at a regionally accredited United States college or university, and a grade of C or better must be earned. An official transcript from the academic institution must accompany the application to take the examination.

If an individual's degree is 10 years old or older, one must meet the current ADA Didactic Program in Dietetics requirements with no fewer than 12 semester- or 18 quarter-hours. A verification statement signed by the program director and a transcript documenting completion of the required courses must be submitted with the examination application. The verification statement must be completed within five years immediately prior to the date of application for registration eligibility.[8]

MAINTAINING REGISTERED STATUS

Continuing education (CE) has always been an integral part of professional registration. CDR was one of the first health credentialing agencies to insist upon continuing education. To maintain registered status, dietetics professionals must acquire 75 hours of approved continuing education every five years.

CDR defines continuing education as education beyond that required for entry into the profession. Educational programs should apply to the field of nutrition and dietetics and should update or enhance one's knowledge and skills in dietetics practice. Some examples of continuing education activities include:

   a. CDR self-assessment modules
   b. Self-study programs
   c. Videotapes of prior-approved educational sessions
   d. Exhibits at trade and educational shows
   e. Poster session attendance
   f. Presentations to professional audiences
   g. Demonstrations related to the field of nutrition and dietetics
   h. Academic coursework

i. Authoring of articles for professional, peer-reviewed publications

j. Study groups and journal clubs.[9]

CDR Self-Assessment Modules

In 1992, CDR made available the first of its self-assessment modules. Self-assessment is a method of continuing professional education that focuses on identifying strengths and needs. The series of modules developed by CDR are designed to help individual practitioners identify their learning needs, make well-informed decisions about how to spend their continuing education time and money, and design a continuing education action plan based on the individual's assessment results.

The modules may be completed at work or at home. They are self-paced, practice-oriented, and approved by CDR for continuing education credits. Modules may include videotape simulation exercises, print materials, case scenarios, or other tools. Questions assess the user's understanding of the concepts and problems presented. After completing a module, it is returned to Pennsylvania State University, Office of Continuing Professional Education to be scored. An individual report is generated and mailed to the module user. Results are totally confidential and available only to the individual dietetic practitioner. The report provides an overall score and a comparison of the module user's score with others' scores, including the scores of other dietetics professionals who share significant professional characteristics. Information on how experts would answer each question and why is also provided. Finally, an action plan worksheet is provided to help the user to map future continuing education goals. Resources for further information on the subject matter are also included.

Module topics include Management, Nutrition Assessment, Nutrition Planning, Nutrition Implementation, Nutrition Evaluation, Nutrition Counseling, Nutrition Programs for Consumers, Managing Financial Resources, Marketing New Products, and Conducting Research. Other modules are scheduled for production in the years ahead.[10]

LICENSURE

Licensure is "a state policy that provides consumers an assurance that a professional is competent to provide certain services and is used by professionals to exclude the nonlicensed from providing those services for a fee. It is a tool for creating and maintaining a verifiable minimum level of skill and competence."[11]

Licensure differs from registration in several ways. While registration is recognized nationally, licensure is recognition by an individual state. Both credentialing systems afford some legal protection to the title of the practitioner, but licensure may also protect the right of an individual to practice in a state. Registration is voluntary, established and maintained in the private sector. Licensure may be either voluntary or mandatory, but has formal legal status in the public sector.

At the present time, 34 states, the District of Columbia, and Puerto Rico have enacted some form of regulation. **Licensing statutes** make it illegal to practice dietetics without first obtaining a license from the state. **Statutory certification** limits the use of particular titles to persons meeting predetermined requirements, but persons not certified can still practice dietetics with a different title. **Registration** is the least restrictive form of state regulation. It prohibits use of the title *dietitian* by persons not meeting state-mandated qualifications. However, unregistered persons may practice the profession.

Each state has a licensure contact person who can provide updates on professional regulation in that state. For the name and telephone number of any state's licensure contact, call the American Dietetic Association at (202)371–0500.

SPECIALITY CERTIFICATION

In 1993, the Commission on Dietetic Registration first offered registered dietitians the opportunity to become board certified specialists in different dietetic specialities. The first three areas of dietetic specialization were renal dietetics, pediatric dietetics, and metabolic nutrition support.

To become a board certified specialist, one must document the following minimum criteria:

- Current registration status and three years minimum length of registration
- 6,000 hours of practice as a registered dietitian in the speciality over the last six years, and current employment of a minimum of 16 hours a week in the speciality area
- successful completion of a practice certification examination

New areas of specialization will be recognized in the coming years. Specialty credentials are also available from other professional organizations. For example, dietitians may become certified diabetes educators (CDE) (a credential offered by the American Diabetes Association) or certified nutrition support dietitians (CNSD) (a credential offered by the American Society for Parenteral and Enteral Nutrition) by meeting the requirements of those organizations.

FELLOW OF THE AMERICAN DIETETIC ASSOCIATION

The American Dietetic Association has established the credential *fellow* to certify those registered dietitians who have demonstrated empirically defined characteristics of achievement and leadership. To become a fellow, candidates must fulfill the following requirements:

- be a registered dietitian
- submit documentation of a minimum of a master's degree, earned and granted by a regionally accred-

ited United States college or university or foreign equivalent

- submit documentation of a minimum of eight years' work experience as a registered dietitian
- submit documentation of at least one professional achievement
- submit documentation of professional positions
- submit documentation of professional contacts
- submit a written response to an approach-to-practice scenario.

A portfolio submitted by the candidate is judged through peer review. Certification as "Fellow of The American Dietetic Association" is granted for a ten-year period. During that period, fellows are required to maintain RD status and submit an annual maintenance fee. At the end of the certification period, fellows who wish to recertify must submit an updated portfolio and a recertification fee.[12]

SUMMARY

Each of you should have the goal of becoming a credentialed dietetics practitioner. While completion of an associate or baccalaureate degree in dietetics is a worthy achievement, it is the earning of the professional credential of D.T.R. or R.D. that opens doors for successful professional practice. This credential is customers' assurance of your qualifications to practice, and it indicates that you actively work to update yourself on the latest information about food and nutrition issues. Licensure indicates that the state in which you practice recognizes your professional competence and expertise.

Specialty certification will become more common in the years ahead, as dietetics practice becomes increasingly complex and diverse. Recognition of leadership and exceptional practice in dietetics by attaining the Fellow of the ADA credential is a goal to which all students in dietetics should aspire. Professional credentialing is the mark of quality practice; it assures the public that the dietetic technician or registered dietitian is providing the highest quality in dietetics services.

SUGGESTED ACTIVITIES

1. Talk to someone who has recently taken the registration examination for dietitian or dietetic technician. What was their reaction to the experience? What suggestions do they have for preparing for the exam?

2. Who is your state continuing education coordinator? If possible, talk to this individual and find out what kinds of continuing education events he/she approves. What process must be followed to get an event approved for continuing education credit?

3. Attend a continuing education event with a dietetics professional, faculty member, or another student. What kind of documentation must be provided for an attendee to receive continuing education credits?

4. Find out if your state has licensure for dietitians. If so, invite someone to your class to talk about licensure, what it means in your state, and how it was obtained in the legislature. What is the process for becoming licensed in your state?

NOTES

1. *Webster's New Universal Unabridged Dictionary.* 2nd ed. New York: Simon and Schuster; 1983.

2. Webster's New Universal Unabridged Dictionary.

3. Woodward NM. *The past, present, and future of dietetics credentialing.* Future Search Conference: Challenging the Future of Dietetic Education and Credentialing. Background Papers. Chicago: The American Dietetic Association and The Commission on Dietetic Registration, Chicago: June 12–14, 1994.

4. Webster's New Universal Unabridged Dictionary.

5. Commission on Dietetic Registration of The American Dietetic Association, personal communication, October 10, 1994.

6. Commission on Dietetic Registration, personal communication.

7. *Components of the Certification Testing Program.* Chicago: The Commission on Dietetic Registration; 1989.

8. *1994 Desk Reference for Educators.* Chicago: Commission on Dietetic Registration; 1994.

9. *Continuing Professional Education. Guidelines for the Registered Dietitian.* Chicago: Commission on Dietetic Registration; 1991.

10. *Self-Assessment: A New Approach to Continuing Professional Education.* Chicago: Commission on Dietetic Registration; 1992.

11. Licensure of dietitians and nutritionists: Update on state laws. *Journal of the American Dietetic Association*, 1994;94:974.

12. *Fellow of the American Dietetic Association.* Chicago: Commission on Dietetic Registration; 1994.

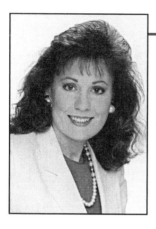

Susan Mitchell

Practicalories™
Maitland, Florida

When I headed off to the University of Tennessee and majored in home economics, I was sure of one thing—my career and my focus would not be traditional. I learned about dietetics as a career after arriving at UT with an undeclared major. My Dad had just been put on a low-cholesterol diet, and he told me about the R.D. who had instructed him and that there was a nutrition program at UT. I was always fascinated with the medical field, but more from the aspect of staying healthy. Wellness has suited me perfectly!

After graduating from the coordinated program in dietetics at UT, I went on to complete both master's and doctoral degrees. I moved to Florida, where my career started out traditionally—I worked part-time at a hospital and consulted for nursing homes and alcohol rehab centers. However, I knew I was not cut out to be in traditional dietetics. I've always had an entrepreneurial spirit, and I put that to use to create, along with my partner Dorine Smith, a business called Practicalories™.

The main focus of the business is to provide consulting, speaking, media, and writing services to corporations, conventions, and food companies. We have been fortunate to work with radio and television for more than four years, providing fun and informative nutrition segments for the public. Our projects vary from consulting for police and fire departments, to writing computer-based training courses, to consulting with food companies on the introduction of new products. The services we provide force us to stay current with the latest trends in nutrition and food.

Another activity I enjoy is organizing grocery store tours to teach individuals how to be smart consumers and purchase healthy foods. I also have a talk show on WDBO in Orlando during morning drive time to bring practical nutrition information to business people. I have a television show at noon that caters to retired individuals and stay-at-home moms. The listening audience for these media offerings is approximately 350,000 people every day!

Dietetics has finally come into its own in terms of importance. My favorite thing about dietetics is that its opportunities are limited only by your own imagination and creativity. My biggest frustration is the image and pay of R.D.s in health-care facilities. Our training and financial value far exceed the current pay scale.

If I could offer words of wisdom to future practitioners, it would be this: don't be afraid to dream and reach for goals outside the normal paradigm. Take elective courses when possible in areas of business management, finance, exercise physiology, or psychology to further expand your knowledge in your chosen area of interest.

CHAPTER 7

◆

The Dietetic Team

M embers of the dietetic team can most often be found working in the institutional healthcare setting. Dietitians, dietetic technicians, and dietary managers are the primary positions that make up the dietetic team. In recent years, healthcare issues such as labor shortages, cost containment, and quality assurance have forced the dietetic team to be better coordinated and to delegate less specialized, more routine tasks to less highly trained personnel.

Members of the dietetic team receive formal training in nutrition and foods. The demand for personnel with this background is greater than the supply. The number of employment opportunities continues to expand. A wide variety of settings for such work exists, and the responsibilities encompassed by each job are as varied as the settings.

MEMBERS OF THE TEAM

The Dietitians

Dietitians are highly qualified professionals who are recognized experts on food and nutrition. The educational requirements to become a dietitian were described in Chapter 3. The American Dietetic Association (ADA) is the primary professional association for dietitians and dietetic technicians. Dietitians work in a wide variety of settings, most of which fall into seven major categories:

Business Dietitians. Business dietitians work in areas such as food manufacturing, advertising, and marketing. Dietitians who work for food manufacturers or grocery chains may analyze the nutrition content of foods for labeling purposes or marketing efforts. They may also prepare literature for distribution to customers and write articles for the news media. In order to satisfy consumers' growing interest in nutrition, dietitians are employed by businesses to develop new products, sell and market products, and develop public relations and advertising programs. Many entrepreneurial dietitians have developed a product, product line, or a service themselves, and built a company to market and sell the products or services.

Clinical Dietitians. Clinical dietitians provide nutritional services for patients in hospitals, nursing homes, clinics, health maintenance organizations, doctors' offices, and other healthcare facilities. They assess patients' nutritional needs, develop and implement nutrition programs, and evaluate and report the results. They are a vital part of the healthcare team, working with doctors and other healthcare professionals to coordinate nutritional intake with other treatment such as medications.

Many clinical dietitians specialize in one area of practice. Diabetes, heart disease, pediatrics, gerontology, kidney disease, the critically ill, and obesity are some of the areas in which clinical dietitians specialize. Nutritional care of the critically ill, for example, involves overseeing the preparation of custom-mixed, high-nutrition formulas for patients requiring tube or intravenous feedings. Clinical dietitians working with diabetics teach patients how to establish and adhere to a long-term nutrition program and how to monitor blood glucose levels.

In addition to assessing nutrition needs and developing treatment plans, clinical dietitians have administrative and managerial duties. The clinical dietitian in a small nursing home or hospital may run the foodservice department. In larger facilities, clinical dietitians may supervise dietetic technicians and other support staff such as patient service supervisors, diet clerks, and clerical personnel.

Community Dietitians. Community dietitians reach out to the public to teach, monitor, and advise individuals and groups in their efforts to prevent disease and promote good health. They are employed by international organizations; federal, state and local governments; food businesses; and trade associations. A variety of public, private, and volunteer organizations concerned with international health employ community nutritionists. The United Nations and the Peace Corps are just two such organizations. The U.S. Department of Agriculture, U.S. Department of Health and Human Services, and the public health division of state and local governments employ community nutritionists to plan and carry out programs to address nutritional problems of targeted groups. The WIC program is one example. The main responsibility of community nutritionists employed by food businesses and associations is nutrition education. Large-scale nutrition education programs for school children and other groups have been organized by the dairy industry, for example. (See Figure 7.1.)

Community dietitians evaluate individual needs, establish nutritional care plans, and communicate the principles of good nutrition in a way individuals and their families can understand. Teaching is a very large component of the community dietitian's job. Topics run the gamut from grocery shopping to the preparation of infant formula, from menu planning for diabetics to alcoholism, from breastfeeding to hypertension.

Consultant Dietitians. Consultant dietitians may be self-employed in their own private practice or under contract to one or more healthcare facilities. In private practice, the consultant dietitian performs nutrition

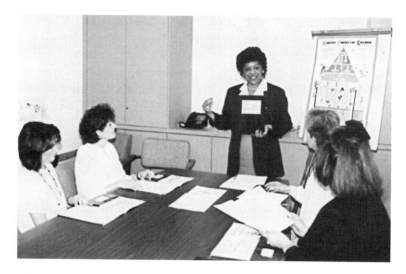

Figure 7.1
A dairy council dietitian conducts a nutrition education program.

screening and assessment of clients, who are often referred by a physician. Weight loss is the most common diet-related concern of clients who seek a private practice dietitian. Consultant dietitians under contract to healthcare facilities provide expert advice on food-service management issues such as menu planning, budgeting, cost control, portion control, sanitation, and safety as well as monitor clinical nutritional care (Figure 7.2).

Educator Dietitians. Educator dietitians teach future dietitians, dietetic technicians, dietary managers, doctors, nurses, dentists, chefs, and others the science of foods and nutrition. They are employed by universities, four-year colleges, community colleges, technical schools, and dietetic internship programs. Although education is a major component of most dietitians' job responsibilities, this category is for those who are employed by an educational institution or program, rather than an organization whose primary responsibility is healthcare.

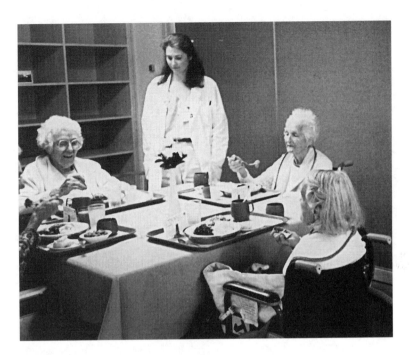

Figure 7.2
A consultant dietitian checking a meal service.

Management Dietitians. Management dietitians play a very important role wherever food is served. They are responsible for large-scale meal planning and preparation in such places as hospitals, nursing homes and retirement residences, company cafeterias, correctional facilities, elementary and secondary schools, food factories, colleges and universities, transportation companies, restaurants, the military, and recreational facilities.

The management dietitian supervises the planning, preparation, and service of meals; selects, trains, and directs other dietitians, foodservice supervisors, and foodservice workers; budgets for and purchases food, equipment, and supplies; enforces sanitary and safety regulations; and prepares records and reports (Figure 7.3).

Dietitians who direct food and nutrition departments also decide on departmental policies and coordinate food

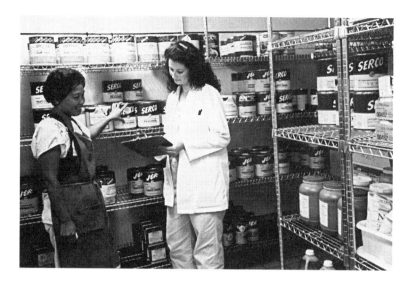

Figure 7.3
A management dietitian at work.

and nutrition services with the activities of other departments. The use of computer programs to adjust recipes, prepare purchase orders, cost recipes and menus, keep inventory records, prepare financial reports, conduct nutritional analyses, etc., has simplified many of the routine functions of management dietetics.

Research Dietitians. Research dietitians work for government agencies, food and pharmaceutical companies, academic medical centers, or educational institutions. Using the scientific method and analytical techniques, they conduct studies that range from pure to applied science. Often research is conducted collaboratively with physicians, exercise physiologists, chemists, food technologists, and researchers from other disciplines. Research dietitians may explore the way the body uses a particular food or the interaction of drugs and diet. They may investigate the nutritional needs of individuals with different diseases or ways to reduce the risk of disease. Research in the managerial arena may involve the effectiveness of various foodservice systems or the efficiency of different types of foodservice equipment.

Dietetic Technicians

Dietetic technicians complete a two-year associate degree in an ADA-approved dietetic technician program that combines both classroom and supervised practice experiences. They are then eligible to take the registration examination for dietetic technicians. Individuals who pass the exam may then use the initials *D.T.R.*, for *Dietetic Technician, Registered*, after their names.

D.T.s work in a wide variety of settings and assume an even-wider variety of responsibilities. D.T.s are found in hospitals, public health nutrition programs, long-term care facilities, child nutrition and school lunch programs, nutrition programs for the elderly, and foodservice management. Screening patients to identify nutritional problems, modifying menus, providing patient education and counseling to individuals and groups, developing menus and recipes, supervising foodservice personnel, purchasing food, conducting inventory, and maintaining computer systems are the most commonly performed functions of a dietetic technician.

Dietary Managers

Dietary managers are members of the Dietary Managers Association (DMA). While no legal relationship exists between the ADA and the DMA, a very close working relationship has always been in existence. Educational requirements, job settings and responsibilities, and the DMA were described in detail in Chapter 4.

SPECIALTY AREAS AND NEW EMPLOYMENT OPPORTUNITIES

Here is a listing of some of the employment opportunities related to nutrition and foods:

Clinical dietitian
Commercial foodservice administrator

Community college educator

Consulting nutritionist

Consumer and public relations specialist for food companies

Diet counselor

Educational representative for business

Extension service 4H coordinator

Extension service home advisor

Food advertising consultant

Food analyst/technologist

Food broker

Food editor

Food journalist

Food photography specialist

Food quality assurance specialist

Food research and marketing specialist

Food scientist

Food science educator

Foodservice administrator for airlines or cruise line

Food stylist

Home economist for food or equipment business

Hospital foodservice administrator

Marketing specialist for food and nutrition companies

Nutrition educator

Nutrition researcher

Peace Corps representative

Private practice

Product development researcher

Public health nutritionist

Rehabilitation consultant

Research chemist

Restaurant foodservice administrator

Sales representative for food or equipment

School foodservice administrator

Sports nutritionist

Taste panel coordinator

Test kitchen scientist[1]

This list is by no means exhaustive, but it shows the breadth of opportunities that are available to someone who has training in foods and nutrition.

DIETETIC PRACTICE GROUPS

Because of the increasingly specialized nature of dietetic practice, the leadership of ADA developed Dietetic Practice Groups (DPGs). DPGs provide a way for members of ADA to network within their area or areas of interest and practice. Currently, there are 25 DPGs, and members of ADA may join as many DPGs as they desire. Dues are paid annually when ADA dues are paid. Dues vary from $10 to $25 a year.

DPG membership affords a member the following opportunities:

- to increase knowledge in a specific area of dietetic practice through newsletters, publications, and continuing education;
- to develop, sponsor, and/or attend workshops and seminars for continuing education credit at the ADA Annual Meeting and throughout the year;
- to develop legislative and public policy materials for ADA;
- to contribute technical expertise to ADA;
- to establish activities that market the profession in general and the practice area in particular; and
- to provide guidelines for practice and quality assurance materials to help practitioners provide a high level of care.

At the present time, the following practice groups are functioning:

DPG–10 Public Health Nutrition. Local, state, and federal government nutrition professionals who work with all age groups in the public health arena

DPG–11 Gerontological Nutritionists. Practitioners who provide and manage nutrition programs and services to older adults in a variety of settings: community, homebound, healthcare facilities, education, and research

DPG–12 Dietetics in Developmental and Psychiatric Disorders. Nutrition professionals whose work involves clients with physical and mental disabilities, developmental disorders, psychiatric illnesses, substance abuse, and eating disorders

DPG–14 Vegetarian Nutrition. Nutrition professionals in community, clinical, education, or foodservice settings who wish to learn about plant-based diets and provide support to individuals following a vegetarian lifestyle

DPG–15 Hunger and Malnutrition. Practitioners working toward public policies that reduce domestic and local hunger and malnutrition and practitioners who work in federal food programs or private programs such as food banks or shelters

DPG–20 Oncology Nutrition. Nutrition professionals who are involved in the care of cancer patients, cancer prevention, and cancer research

DPG–21 Renal Dietitians. Practitioners who work in dialysis facilities, clinics, hospitals, and private-practice renal nutrition counseling

DPG–22 Pediatric Nutrition. Practitioners who provide nutrition services for the pediatric population in a wide variety of settings

DPG–23 Diabetes Care and Education. Practitioners involved in patient education, professional education, or research for the management of diabetes mellitus

DPG–24 Dietitians in Nutrition Support. Practitioners integrating the science of enteral and parenteral nutrition to provide appropriate nutrition support to individuals in inpatient and outpatient settings

DPG–25 Dietetics in Physical Medicine and Rehabilitation. Practitioners who provide nutrition support, counseling, and education to clients undergoing rehabilitation in inpatient/outpatient centers, group homes, transitional living centers, and industry

DPG–27 Dietitians in General Clinical Practice. Practitioners who possess a mosaic of professional skills, who provide and/or manage nutrition care in settings ranging from acute to long term, and who maintain working knowledge in many clinical areas

DPG–30 Consulting Nutritionists. Entrepreneurial practitioners in the business of developing and delivering nutrition-related services and/or products—membership ranges from veteran business owners to members establishing new practices

DPG–31 Consultant Dietitians in Health Care Facilities. Practitioners, typically employed under contract, who provide nutrition consultation to acute and long-term care facilities, home care companies, healthcare agencies, and the foodservice industry

DPG–32 Dietitians in Business and Communications. Professionals employed by, seeking employment in, or self-employed in the profit-making organizations of the food and nutrition industry

DPG–33 Sports and Cardiovascular Nutritionists. Nutrition professionals with expertise and skills in promoting the role of nutrition in physical performance, cardiovascular health, and wellness

DPG–41 ADA Members with Management Responsibilities in Healthcare Delivery Systems. Food and nutrition care managers generally employed in institutions—includes directors of departments or facilities and administrative dietitians and technicians

DPG–42 School Nutrition Services. Food and nutrition care managers employed by school feeding programs, and directors of the child nutrition programs of these operations

DPG–43 Dietitians in College and University Food Service. Food and nutrition care managers who direct operations in colleges and universities

DPG–44 Clinical Nutrition Management. Managers who direct clinical nutrition programs in healthcare settings

DPG–45 Technical Practice in Dietetics. Dietetic technicians, dietetic technician educators, and dietetic technician employers who focus on the competencies, skills, and needs of dietetic technicians

DPG–50 Dietetic Educators of Practitioners. Educators of students enrolled in dietetic technician programs, didactic programs in dietetics, coordinated programs, approved preprofessional practice programs (AP4s), dietetic internships, and other programs

DPG–51 Nutrition Educators of Health Professionals. Members invited or involved in education and communication with physicians, nurses, dentists, and other healthcare professionals

DPG–52 Nutrition Education for the Public. Practitioners involved in the design, implementation, and evaluation of nutrition education programs for target populations

DPG–54 Nutrition Research. Members who conduct research in the various areas of practice and are employed in the different practice settings of dietetics[2]

PRACTICE AWARDS

A number of awards for excellence in practice are given annually by the ADA and by affiliated state associations of ADA. The current ADA awards and honors are:

Marjorie Hulsizer Copher Award. The highest honor bestowed upon a member of the ADA.

Lenna Frances Cooper Memorial Lecturer. Given annually to a member who reflects the high standards and ideals personified by Miss Cooper, a pioneer in the ADA (Figure 7.4). She proposed its formation, cofounded and chaired the first National Conference of Dietitians, and served as first vice-president and fourteenth president.

Outstanding State Professional Recruitment Coordinator (SPRC). Recognizes dietetics professionals who have successfully developed, coordinated, and

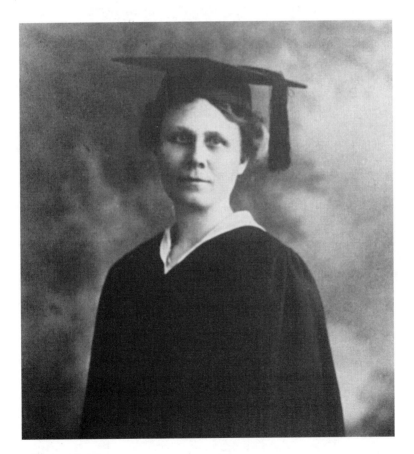

Figure 7.4
Lenna Frances Cooper, founding member.
Photo courtesy of The American Dietetic Association.

participated in their state affiliate's student recruitment network.

Medallion Awards. Recognize five members who have made significant contributions to the professional association and the profession in general.

Awards for Excellence. Recognize RDs who have demonstrated leadership in the profession through innovative practice, participation in educational and networking events, and sharing of professional information to increase the knowledge of dietetics professionals. These awards are given in the areas of Clinical Nutrition, Community Dietetics, Consultation and Private Practice, Management Practice, Dietetic Education, and Dietetic Research.

Anita Owen Recognition Award for Innovative Nutrition Education Programs for the Public. Encourages the development of, and recognizes excellence in, innovative and unique models for dietetic information and/or services for delivery of nutrition education to the public.

Honorary Membership. Awarded to nonmembers who have demonstrated active promotion and support for the profession of dietetics and/or the sound nutrition principles for which it stands.

New Researcher's Award. Recognizes the work of a new researcher in the field.

Media Excellence Award. Recognizes the work of a member of the media for his/her contributions in reporting food and nutrition information to the American public.

Judy Ford Stokes Award for Innovation in Administrative Dietetics or Foodservice Facility Design. Encourages further development of administrative dietetics through cost-effective methods and/or revenue-generating techniques in foodservice facility design.

Huddleson Award. Honors a registered dietitian who was the lead author of a peer-reviewed article, published in the *Journal of the American Dietetic Association* during the previous calendar year, that made an important contribution to the dietetics profession.

Distinguished Service Awards. Bestowed upon members of the United States Congress who have demonstrated outstanding service and support on nutrition and health issues of importance to the Association and to the public.

President's Circle Nutrition Education Award. Recognizes the development and dissemination of scientifically sound nutrition information that is unique, creative, unusual in approach, and free from specific commercial endorsement.

Instructional Award for Excellence in Affirmative Action. Recognizes the significant accomplishments of an ADA-accredited/approved dietetic education program in increasing and improving recruitment, selection, and support of ethnic minorities and male students.

Council on Practice, Dietetic Practice Group Awards. Include the following:

- Gerontological Nutritionists DPG Joncier Greene Continuing Education Award
- Pediatric Nutrition DPG Published Research Award
- Pediatric Nutrition DPG Outstanding Member Award
- Pediatric Nutrition DPG Creative Nutrition Education Award
- Sports and Cardiovascular Nutritionist DPG Achievement Award
- Nutrition Research DPG Published Paper—First Author Award
- Nutrition Research DPG Published Paper—Contributing Author Award
- Nutrition Research DPG New Investigator Award

STANDARDS OF PRACTICE

The ADA House of delegates approved Standards of Practice in 1984 after more than four years of work. These Standards outline a dietetic practitioner's responsibilities for providing quality nutritional care. The standards provide individual practitioners with a systematic plan for implementing, evaluating, and adjusting performance in any area of practice.

Standard 1: The dietetic practitioner establishes performance criteria, compares actual performance with expected performance, documents results, and takes appropriate action.

Standard 2: The dietetic practitioner develops, implements, and evaluates an individual plan for practice based on assessment of consumer needs, current knowledge, and clinical experience.

Standard 3: The dietetic practitioner, utilizing unique knowledge of nutrition, collaborates with other professionals, personnel, and/or consumers in integrating, interpreting, and communicating nutrition care principles.

Standard 4: The dietetic practitioner engages in life-long self-development to improve knowledge and skills.

Standard 5: The dietetic practitioner generates, interprets, and uses research to enhance dietetic practice.

Standard 6: The dietetic practitioner identifies, monitors, analyzes, and justifies the use of resources.[3]

Each standard is specifically defined by specific criteria. For example, Standard 4, Criteria 1 states, "Conduct self-assessment to identify professional strengths and weaknesses."

ROLE DELINEATION STUDIES

In order to identify the major and specific responsibilities that dietetic practitioners must assume to ensure quality care, the ADA conducts role delineation studies. Three studies, conducted in 1983 and 1984, focused on what practitioners in clinical dietetics, community dietetics, and foodservice systems management were doing and what they ought to be doing.[4] A 1990 study measured what practitioners in a variety of settings actually do, at entry-level and beyond. No measures of quality, correctness, or efficacy were included in the 1990 study. The results of the study are not being used just to define appropriate responsibilities and knowledge-bases for competent dietetic practice. The educational component of the profession will use the data collected to update knowledge and performance requirements and develop curriculum. The practice component of the profession will use the study to revise practice standards and develop outcome criteria for quality assurance. And the certification component of the profession will use the study as a basis for test specifications for the registration examinations.[5]

SUMMARY

Dietitians, dietetic technicians, and dietary managers are the members of the dietetic team. They have all received formal training in foods and nutrition and, as a team, work in a wide variety of settings. Dietitians, who are recognized experts in food and nutrition, are found working in the business, clinical, community, consulting, education, management, and research arenas. Dietetic technicians must complete a two-year associate degree in an ADA-approved dietetic technician program and then pass the registration examination for Dietetic Technicians. Dietary managers complete a one-year college course.

The American Dietetic Association has developed Dietetic Practice Groups to allow members to network and increase their knowledge within their particular area of practice; annual awards for excellence in specific areas of practice; and standards of practice which outline a dietetic practitioner's responsibilities for providing quality nutritional care.

SUGGESTED ACTIVITIES

1. Choose one of the dietetic practice groups you might be interested in joining later in your career. If possible, attend one of the meetings of this practice group at an annual meeting of ADA or at a regional meeting. Or, interview a member of the practice group to find out what the practice group does to benefit the profession and individual members.

2. Contact a large medical center or hospital in your area to see if a dietetic team is present. Talk to the members of the team to determine their roles and responsibilities in delivering nutritional care to clients.

3. With a team of fellow students, write a paper on the principles of teamwork. In doing the research and writing the paper, apply the principles that have been found to be effective. Evaluate your success as a team. What worked well and why? What didn't work and why?

4. Add to the list of specialty areas of dietetic practice included in the chapter by either listing positions you know exist or by developing areas of practice or positions you would be interested in personally. Be creative!

NOTES

1. American Dietetic Association. *Set Your Sights: Your Future in Dietetics*. Chicago: The American Dietetic Association; 1991.

2. American Dietetic Association. *Dietetic Practice Groups*. Chicago: The American Dietetic Association; 1994.

3. Standards of practice for the profession of dietetics. *Journal of the American Dietetic Association*, 1985;85:723–726.

4. American Dietetic Association. *Role Delineation and Verification for Entry-Level Positions in Community Dietetics*. Chicago: The American Dietetic Association; 1983. American Dietetic Association. *Role Delineation and Verification for Entry-Level Positions in Food Service Systems Management*. Chicago: The American Dietetic Association; 1983. American Dietetic Association. *Role Delineation and Verification for Entry-Level Positions in Clinical Dietetics*. Chicago: The American Dietetic Association; 1984.

5. American Dietetic Association. *Role Delineation for Registered Dietitians and Entry-Level Dietetic Technicians*. Chicago: The American Dietetic Association; 1990.

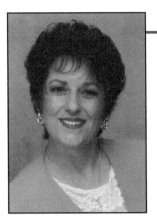

Penny Walters

*Springhouse Assisted Living
Boynton Beach, Florida*

In 1984, I enrolled in a computer technology course to retool for a new career. After just one semester, I realized that computer technology was *not* for me. While looking through the course catalog, dietetics jumped out at me—it was a blend of all things I held near and dear to my heart. Having done catering and bookkeeping most of my life, and having a keen interest in healthy eating, dietetics was right up my alley.

I changed my major, and enrolled in the dietetic technician program at Palm Beach Community College. My two clinical practicums were done at local hospitals and a management practicum was done at a local nursing home. I graduated in May, 1987, and became one of the first dietetic technicians to become registered by sitting for the credentialing exam— having graduated one semester too late to be grandfathered in!

After graduation, I decided to pursue a career in management and began my own consulting business. My clients included various adult congregate living facilities, weight loss programs, local hospitals needing vacation relief, a local "fat farm" which needed someone to oversee food preparation, and Palm Beach Community College, where I taught basic food preparation and nutrition classes.

Having a consulting business allowed me time for involvement with the professional association. I was honored to be named Florida Dietetic Technician of the Year in 1988.

In 1989 I founded a support group and job bank for technicians in the Palm Beach area. This was a great support and networking opportunity, especially for new technicians coming into the area. In 1990, and again in 1993 I accepted positions in the foods and nutrition departments of hospitals and long-term care facilities in need of guidance and structure. In both instances, my education and training served me well, enabling me and the staff to reduce turnover, increase customer satisfaction, and come in under budget. With the support of a wonderful consultant dietitian, I was able to ease back into clinical dietetic practice, learning about the new federal Medicare guidelines and other changes which had occurred in clinical practice.

A year ago I accepted a position as regional director of foodservice systems for Springhouse Assisted Living. On any given day, long-term care residents interact with the foodservice department more than any other department in the facility. I work closely with the corporate dietitians who provide assistance with menus, forms, and systems. It has been exciting to oversee the foodservice operations of the twelve Springhouse facilities and our division continues to grow.

I have been very fortunate, over the past nine years, to have support and assistance of my mentor, Ethel Fowler, and consultant RDs. I have been able to perform my job duties as described, and I'm very proud to say I'm a registered dietetic technician.

CHAPTER 8

---◆---

The Healthcare Team

L ong gone are the days of the family doctor acting alone to treat disease. A career in healthcare is no longer limited to being either a doctor or nurse. The healthcare system in the United States is one of the most sophisticated and complex in the world. The increase in number of elderly people (there are now three million more people over the age of 75 than there were five years ago); rampant shortages in the health-care workforce; specialized treatments requiring complex technology; increasing emphasis on preventive healthcare; and an increased understanding of the cost benefits of a healthy workforce all create very positive prospects for anyone entering a healthcare career.

Prevailing economic conditions appear to have no impact on the outlook for healthcare careers. In the past ten years, three million jobs have been created in healthcare. During a ten-month period in the early 1990s, the total U.S. economy lost 1.4 million jobs, while healthcare services grew by 390,000 new jobs.

The explosion of knowledge in science has led to a corresponding explosion in the number of healthcare professions that demand specialized knowledge and skills. The term *allied health* is used to describe a cluster of roles in the healthcare system that assist, facilitate, and complement the work of physicians and other healthcare specialists. For example, the data acquired by laboratory technicians plays a crucial role in the detection, diagnosis, and treatment of disease. The medical records administrator collects, analyzes, and manages information that steers the healthcare industry. The rehabilitation process for a patient often requires the combined efforts of physical therapists, a medical social worker, occupational therapists, and dietitians. The hospital pharmacist works with nurses, doctors, and dietitians to provide quality patient care. These specialty areas free highly skilled medical practitioners to perform the tasks they alone are qualified to do.

Along with the expansion in number of allied health professions, there has been an expansion in the number of work settings. Fitness centers, gyms, and spas are examples of nontraditional settings where dietitians are finding employment today.

Almost eight million people are employed in health service careers, according to the U.S. Department of Labor. By the end of the 1990s, it is estimated that this figure will rise to 12 million or more.[1] The American Society of Allied Health Professions lists more than 85 different health service careers.[2]

The high demand, combined with stability, excellent starting salaries, mobility, and flexibility make a health services career very attractive to those with the desire to help others. The attributes and skills that are considered characteristic of successful healthcare professionals are: enjoyment of the basic biological sciences; intellectual capacity to solve problems; flexibility; patience; investigative skills; respect for others as human beings; effective communication skills; counseling skills; diagnostic and teaching skills; research design skills; computer skills; an understanding of technical equipment; and the ability to be a team player.

The concept of the team approach in the healthcare setting, encompassing a number of health professionals, has been increasingly encouraged in the past 25 years in order to provide patients/clients with safe, timely, and effective care.

THE HISTORY OF THE HEALTHCARE TEAM CONCEPT

The concept of the healthcare team emerged after World War II with an increased social awareness and expectations of healthcare for all. Disabled veterans returning from the war needed more than traditional medical treatment for their physical disabilities: they needed all kinds of help in order to return to the community as socially and economically useful citizens. The trend toward sharing responsibilities that had formerly been the sole purview of the physician and/or nurse has had a major impact on quality of care, healthcare costs, and the organization and delivery of healthcare.[3]

TEAMWORK

Teamwork is the close, cooperative effort of several people to use their special skills and knowledge to meet the needs of the client/patient more efficiently, completely, competently, and considerately than would be possible by individual, independent action.[4] An important, but often forgotten, member of the team is the client/patient. Educating and including the client/patient in the team communication process is critically important.[5] Because the ultimate responsibility for client/patient care rests with the physician, it is the physician who assumes leadership of most healthcare teams. Other members of the team vary depending on the needs of the client/patient.

In order to function effectively, healthcare teams must be able to differentiate between those roles that are unique to each discipline and those that are shared. Team members function independently when they have unique competencies, knowledge, and experiences. Delegated functioning occurs when the team has varying levels and types of training. Collaborative functioning is utilized when an overlap in competencies allows for a common base for judgment and decision-making.[6]

A clinical dietitian doing a patient discharge diet instruction is functioning independently. A delegated function for this same dietitian would be the implementation of a physician-prescribed diet order. An example of a collaborative, multidisciplinary approach would be the implementation of a weight-control program involving a physician, dietitian, exercise physiologist, laboratory technician, and psychologist.[7] Diseases that have systemic effects are natural candidates for the collaborative, multidisciplinary team approach. For example care for diabetic patients, often involves a primary care physician, endocrinologist, dietitian, nurse/nurse practitioner, ophthalmologist, podiatrist, health educator, and others.

Teamwork may be problematic if roles are not clearly defined, communication is not adequate and open, members fail to be good team players, and team goals are not clearly defined. Accurate and timely sharing of data is a key element in the effectiveness of the team effort. Team conferences, where all team members share information and participate in decision making, are the preferred approach.

MEMBERS OF THE HEALTHCARE TEAM

There are more than 85 possible members of the healthcare team! A few are highlighted in the following section.

Physicians

Required training includes a four-year postgraduate medical degree (either an M.D. or a D.O.). Medical schools in the United States have specific undergraduate entrance requirements including mathematics, sciences, and humanities. Entrance to medical school is very competitive and based on undergraduate GPA, the results of a standardized medical school entrance exam, letters of recommendation, and community service, volunteer, or research experience.

Medical school includes two years of basic medical science followed by two years of clinical training. The clinical training concentrates heavily on the daily care of hospitalized patients. During these two years medical students begin to explore areas of specialization in medicine. Following graduation from medical school, most doctors complete a residency in a specialty, which lasts three to five years. A fellowship may follow the residency program if a doctor wants to train in a subspecialty area. For example, a residency in pediatrics could be followed by a fellowship in neonatology (care of newborns including premature infants), pediatric cardiology (the heart and circulatory system), pediatric neurology (the brain and nervous system), pediatric hematology (the blood), pediatric oncology (cancer and tumors), pediatric gastroenterology (the digestive system), or pediatric nephrology (the kidneys).

A primary care physician provides the majority of care to well and sick patients. The primary care specialties are pediatrics (infants and children), family practice, geriatrics (the elderly) and obstetrics/gynecology. Other physician specialties are listed here.

Cardiologists. Cardiologists diagnose and treat cardiovascular defects and diseases. They are concerned with structure and function of the heart and blood vessels and with the circulation of blood throughout the body.

Oncologists. Oncology is concerned with neoplastic growth (abnormal new growth of cells and tissues), including the cause and the pattern of the abnormality.

Neurologists. Neurology is an internal medicine specialty that deals with disorders of the human brain, spinal cord, peripheral nerves, and muscles. Neurologists care for patients with a myriad of disorders such as pain, weakness in arms or legs, or memory loss.

Pathologists. Pathologists provide and interpret laboratory information to help solve diagnostic problems and monitor the effects of therapy for other medical specialists.

Endocrinologists. An endocrinologist diagnoses and treats diseases of the hormone-producing glandular system, including the pituitary, thyroid, parathyroid, adrenals, and gonads and the insulin-producing cells of the pancreas. Endocrinologists also treat patients with metabolic disorders.

Surgeons. Surgeons deal with problems by using operative procedures. The problems may be mechanical or structural (such as hernias, fractures, or ulcers); biological (such as an ulcer); or metabolic (such as an islet cell tumor of the pancreas, which causes the pancreas to secrete too much insulin). Surgical subspecialties include: gastrointestinal (digestive tract), plastic surgery, vascular (blood vessels), cardiothoracic (heart and chest), pediatric (children), endocrine (glands), orthopedic (bones and joints), urology (kidney and bladder), neurologic (brain and nervous system), otolaryngology (ear, nose, and throat), gynecology (female organs), hand, trauma and burn, oncology (cancer), and transplantation (transplanted organs).

Psychiatrists. Psychiatrists treat patients with mental illnesses and are able to prescribe medicines for illnesses such as depression and schizophrenia.

Podiatrists. Podiatrists specialize in the care and treatment of the human foot.

Ophthalmologists. Ophthalmology is the branch of medicine dealing with the structure, function, and diseases of the eye, including medical and surgical treatment of its defects and diseases.

Osteopathic Physicians. Osteopathy is a system of medical practice based on a theory that diseases are due chiefly to loss of structural integrity which can be restored by manipulation of the parts supplemented by therapeutic measures (such as medicine, physical therapy, or surgery). Osteopathic physicians use the title D.O. which stands for Doctor of Osteopathy.

Chiropractors

A doctor of chiropractic (D.C.) has completed a minimum of two years of college credit toward a baccalaureate degree and three-and-a-half to four years at a chiropractic college. Chiropractic care emphasizes a holistic approach to health, and is based on the premise that the relationship between structure and function in the human body (particularly of the spinal column and nervous system) is a significant health factor. Chiropractors believe that when the spinal column is out of alignment, the body's natural defenses to disease and illness are lowered. Chiropractors realign the spinal column so that the body stays in a state of homeostasis or balance.

Nurses

Nurses are active in the prevention of illness in clinics, industry and public health; the care of patients in emergency and intensive-care situations; general nursing care in hospitals and long-term care settings; and in homes. There are more than 100 nursing specialties. The specialty may focus on a specific disease, organ/system, setting, scope of practice, patient age, criticalness of patient condition, or technology.

Nurse Practitioners. Nurse practitioners are Registered Nurses with advanced formal education. Most have a master's degree in nursing and are certified by a national professional association. Working in collaboration with physicians and other healthcare team members, nurse practitioners obtain medical histories and perform physical exams; diagnose and treat common health problems; diagnose, treat, and monitor chronic diseases; order and interpret lab work and x-rays; prescribe medications and other treatments; provide family planning, prenatal care, well baby and child care, and health maintenance care; conduct patient and family education and counseling programs; provide referrals to healthcare team members; and, in some states, prescribe medicines.

Pharmacists

Hospital pharmacists monitor a patient's drug therapy, prepare intravenous medications and feedings, oversee drug administration, and make purchasing decisions. Pharmacists are an important member of many healthcare teams.

Social Workers

The field of social work is incredibly broad. A bachelor of arts in social work is always required; a master's degree in social work (MSW) is increasingly required. The undergraduate degree is broad-based, with elective courses in substance abuse, grief, and race and gender issues. Graduate programs explore human behavior, mental disorders, and methods of intervention and psychotherapy in greater depth.

Physical Therapists

Physical therapists design and administer rehabilitative exercise programs for people with injuries or disabilities that impact their daily functioning (Figure 8.1).

Athletic Trainers

Athletic trainers provide services such as injury prevention, recognition, immediate care, treatment, and rehabilitation of athletic trauma.

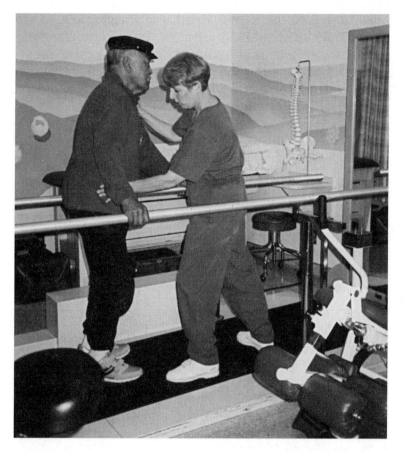

Figure 8.1
A physical therapist assists a stroke patient whose balance and gait have been impaired.

Medical Assistants

Medical assistants assist physicians in their offices or other medical settings by performing a variety of administrative and clinical duties.

Medical Laboratory Technicians/Technologists

Under the supervision of a pathologist, a "lab tech" performs lab tests, using precision instruments, on blood, tissues, and body fluids in order to detect, diagnose, and treat diseases. Medical lab technologists are able to perform the same duties as a technician and can also perform more complex analyses, discrimination, and correction of errors. Histologic technicians/technologists specialize in the preparation of body tissues for laboratory analysis.

Medical Records Administrators

A medical record comprises the complete and permanent documents maintained for every person treated in a medical facility. Medical records administrators manage the medical record in compliance with medical, administrative, ethical, and legal requirements. The medical records technician (MRT) is responsible for maintaining the medical records.

Nuclear Medicine Technologists

A nuclear medicine technologist assists a nuclear medicine physician. These physicians utilize the nuclear properties of radioactive and stable nuclides to make diagnostic evaluations of the anatomic or physiologic conditions of the body.

Occupational Therapists

Occupational therapists and their assistants provide service to individuals whose abilities to cope with the tasks of living are threatened or impaired by developmental deficits, the aging process, poverty and cultural differences, physical injury or illness, or psychological and social disability (Figures 8.2 and 8.3). The therapy is directed toward teaching adaptive skills and enhancing performance capacity in order to achieve optimal function, prevent disability, or maintain health. The goal is the highest possible functional independence for self-care, work, and leisure.

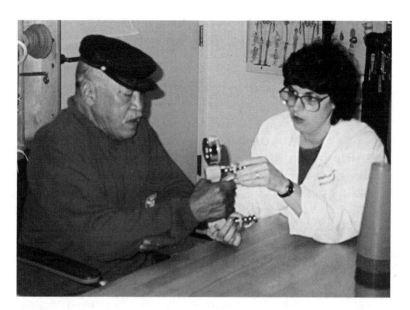

Figure 8.2
An occupational therapist tests a stroke patient's grip.

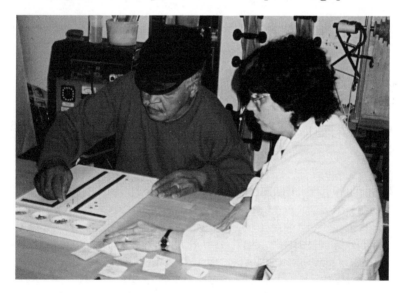

Figure 8.3
Under the watchful eye of an occupational therapist, a stroke patient completes an exercise to improve hand–eye coordination and manual dexterity.

Physician Assistants

The physician assistant (P.A.), under the supervision of a physician, performs diagnostic, therapeutic, preventive, and health maintenance services. Duties include, but are not limited to, the following: performing complete physical examinations; performing and/or interpreting routine diagnostic procedures; giving injections and immunizations; suturing and wound care; and instructing and counseling patients.

Radiologic Technologists

Under the supervision of radiation oncologists, "rad techs" administer radiation therapy to patients. Radiographers, also under the supervision of qualified physicians, provide patient service using imaging modalities.

Respiratory Therapists

The respiratory therapist and respiratory therapy technician evaluate all data to determine the appropriate respiratory care for a patient and conduct the therapeutic procedures to carry out this plan.

SUMMARY

Teamwork is important in the healthcare professions today, due in part to the enormous number of people employed in these careers. In 1990, there were 1,715,600 nurses, 567,611 doctors, 161,900 pharmacists, 60,000 dietitians, and 12,000 podiatrists in the United States. The team approach is an effective way of dealing with the fragmentation of care that may occur due to specialization.

Effective teamwork requires shared goals, clearly defined roles, and a plan for coordinating efforts. Whenever possible, the patient should be part of the team. Any health professional can testify to the importance of patient cooperation in the diagnostic, therapeutic, and rehabilitative processes.

SUGGESTED ACTIVITIES

1. Choose any of the allied health professions. Do an in-depth study of its educational requirements, job responsibilities, areas of specialization, etc.

2. Visit a local hospital cafeteria and talk to as many of its employees as you can. Try to determine if, how, and to what extent they work with members of the dietetic team.

3. Volunteer to work in a hospital or other healthcare facility. This is an excellent way to learn about various healthcare professions and help those who need it at the same time.

NOTES

1. Snelling RO, Snelling AM. *Jobs! What They Are . . . Where They Are . . . What They Pay!*, 3rd ed. New York: Fireside/Simon & Schuster; 1992.

2. Shedlock N. Prognosis for careers in health: Never better. *Journal of Career Planning and Employment*, 1992;52:37–40.

3. Torrens PR. *The American Health Care System: Issues and Problems*. Saint Louis: C.V. Mosby Company; 1978.

4. Pellegrino ED. Interdisciplinary education in the health professions. In: *Educating for the Health Team*. Washington, D.C.: National Academy of Sciences, National Institute of Medicine; 1972. Allen AS, ed. *Introduction to Health Professions*. Saint Louis: C.V. Mosby Company; 1983.

5. Etzweiler DD. The patient is a member of the medical team. *Journal of the American Dietetic Association*, 1972;61:421–423.

6. (a) Modrow CL, Darnell RE. Cross-modality: Delivery of health services through nonprofessionals. *Journal of the American Dietetic Association*, 1979;74:337–340. (b) Modrow CL, Darnell RE. Dietetic services in cross-modality systems. *Journal of the American Dietetic Association*, 1979;74:341–344.

7. Tobias AL, Gordon JB. Social consequences of obesity. *Journal of the American Dietetic Association*, 1980;76:338–342.

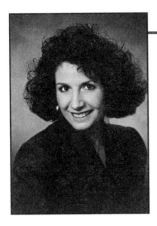

Ann Marie de Jong

Kansas Beef Council
Topeka, Kansas

My name is Ann Marie de Jong, and I am a registered and licensed dietitian from Kansas. You might wonder why I chose to become a dietitian. I actually took three years to narrow my college major, wandering from elementary education, to interior design, to the sciences.

With a little coaxing from some professors, I began the study of dietetics; the more I learned, the more I liked it! Despite the quantity foods laboratory (a little scary for someone who had never even taken a home economics class), I persevered and completed a coordinated program in dietetics at Kansas State University, completing both coursework and practicum experiences simultaneously. Because our program was general in focus, I had the training necessary to practice in foodservice management, clinical dietetics, or community nutrition. In fact, with the growing interest of the public in nutrition, I practically could create my own career!

I have not been disappointed. Dietetics has provided me the opportunity to use my knowledge and creativity in a variety of ways. Following graduation, I worked as a corporate dietitian for a restaurant management company. I was responsible for developing and directing a large-scale nutrition concept to be used in all thirteen of the company's foodservice units. To this end, I developed and analyzed recipes, trained foodservice staff, and evaluated food quality. To ensure that the food coming out of our units was properly prepared and that its preparers were fully aware of the causes and consequences of poor sanitation, I developed a food safety training program known as "The Clean Team."

Through this position, I was also able to promote nutrition awareness on radio, television, and in the print media. One of the most enjoyable aspects of my job was the creation of cooking school programs to showcase the talents of resident and guest chefs. (That quantity foods lab turned out to be worthwhile after all!) Working as a dietitian alongside renowned chefs gave me the satisfaction of knowing that my profession was having an impact in arenas far removed from the typical hospital or institutional foodservice setting. My programs had an impact, not only on the chefs but on everyone who ate the food prepared in their restaurants.

My career has continued to be exciting and varied. I now am Director of Consumer Affairs for the Kansas Beef Council, where I use my knowledge of foods, nutrition, and foodservice management to meet the food and nutrition needs of the public. My degree in dietetics has been practical, valuable (both to myself and others), and, most of all, enjoyable.

CHAPTER 9

◆

Future Trends in Dietetics

If we had a crystal ball and could look into the future, what would we see for the future of dietetics? What roles will dietitians play? What areas of practice, that are unheard of now, will exist in the twenty-first century? What will be the impact of technology on the practice of dietetics? Will the future needs of our clients be different than they are today?

A number of forces and trends are going to reshape the healthcare industry and the practice of dietetics in the coming years. Sara Parks outlines five major forces that will have an impact on the profession of dietetics.[1]

- *Downsizing in hospitals.* Consider the following statistics. From 1980 to 1991, 603 acute-care hospitals and 225 specialty-care facilities closed. In 1992, another 39 hospitals either decreased services or closed completely.[2] Occupancy rates fell more than 7 percent, admissions fell 13.6 percent, and inpatient days decreased 19.5 percent.

- *Emergence of mergers and coalitions.* Mergers and coalitions are means of dealing with skyrocketing costs in healthcare. The growth of these cost-cutting actions is predicted to increase. Such mergers may result in a reduced number of middle-management positions.[3]

- *A shift toward managed care and managed competition.* Managed care and managed competition are two other means of dealing with healthcare costs. Quality of patient services is the overriding goal. New ways of delivering care that make better use of staff expertise and other resources must be developed. Generalist training of dietitians, in management as well as nutrition, should position the dietitian to assume new roles in these care systems.[4]
- *Formation of integrated networks.* Integrated networks mean increased cooperation between hospitals, medical staff, pharmaceutical companies, insurance companies, etc. Increased use of home healthcare and ambulatory care centers is on the horizon in health care.
- *Alterations in referral patterns.* Most insurance companies now require patients to obtain a referral from a primary care physician before seeking the services of an allied health professional. Dietitians must learn to access these physicians and influence these referral systems, in order to be key players on healthcare delivery teams in the future.

In the summer of 1994, the ADA sponsored "The Future Search Conference: Challenging the Future of Dietetic Education and Credentialing," in order to look ahead to these and other issues impacting the future of dietetics. More than 125 participants were selected to represent divergent views and varied areas of practice, education, culture, and geographic location.[5] We don't have a crystal ball, but studying the report of this conference[6] can give us a glimpse of what experts believe is the future of the dietetics profession.

FUTURE PRACTICE ROLES FOR DIETETICS PROFESSIONALS

One of the major factors affecting the future of dietetics will be healthcare reform. While specifics are yet unknown, Congress is likely to enact legislation that will change the current landscape of healthcare in the United States. Dietetics practice can and must evolve as the healthcare environment changes.

One of the speakers for the Future Trends conference was Clemont Bezold, executive director of the Institute for Alternative Futures in Alexandria, Virginia. In his remarks at the conference, Dr. Bezold outlined changes that he believes will impact dietetic practice in the years ahead.[7] These changes include:

- *Genetics and Biochemical Uniqueness.* Understanding the locations and characteristics of specific DNA sequences will give us new information about the workings of our internal "chemical factory" and how our bodies deal with disease. As we learn more and more about the body and its workings, dietitians must be ready to absorb this information and come up with new approaches to diet and foodservice.

- *Nanomedicines and Genetic Foods.* Nanotechnology is the "physical capability of controlling the structure of matter, atom by atom and molecule by molecule." This technology could make possible drugs that could test, diagnose, and repair the human body at the molecular level. Likewise, molecular-level adjustments could be made in the foods we eat, enhancing the nutrition contribution of the food. Dietitians must be prepared to utilize new technologies to advance dietetics practice.

- *Therapeutics and Lifestyle.* New therapies will be developed that will focus on lifestyle factors affecting health and disease; dietary factors are likely to play a major role. Dietitians will be needed to develop the guidelines, implement strategies, and direct the dietary aspects of these new approaches.

- *New Health Care Paradigm: Individual and Community Focus.* In the future, patients will more and more be considered "customers" rather than "cases." According to Dr. Bezold, healthcare providers will play a coaching role, as they help their clients achieve mutually determined health goals. Community health outcomes will gain increasing importance, and healthcare providers will share responsibility for improving these outcomes. Certainly, dietitians will play an important role in both the individual and community focus on health.

- *Smarter Markets.* Dr. Bezold believes that in the future, a public database will make information about healthcare providers available. "Just as the magazine, *Consumer Reports,* now evaluates automobiles and appliances in print, future information systems will provide electronic evaluations of health care providers—including dietitians." Dietitians must be prepared to have their performance objectively critiqued and outcomes of their interventions measured.

- *Reflecting Divergent Values of Consumers.* As consumers better understand the options available to them in the healthcare marketplace, they will be able to make more informed decisions based on their personal value systems. Dietitians must be prepared to incorporate health objectives into various culturally specific diets.

- *Information System Advances.* The use of expert systems to make decisions in healthcare is already being used. New types of expert systems will be developed to deliver dietetic information tailored for various cultural groups, genetic types, or even specific individuals. This specialized information will be available to medical professionals everywhere if they have access to the system. Dietitians must work with those who develop these systems to integrate appropriate clinical knowledge.

- *Home Health Information Systems.* Home health information modules will be available in the future to monitor the health of family members. This monitoring can alert both individuals and their healthcare providers to early indications of many diseases. Dietetic information will be delivered directly to homes, based on age, interest level, knowledge level, and learning style of the recipients. Dietitians should be on the cutting edge of development of such information.

FOODSERVICE TRENDS AND THEIR IMPACT ON FUTURE PRACTICE ROLES

Another participant at the Future Trends conference was Jane Young Wallace, publisher of *Restaurants and Institutions Magazine*. She wrote on the topic "Gateway to the Millennium: How Foodservice Trends Will Impact on Future Practice Roles." Her paper cited 15 areas— beyond the traditional and clinical healthcare sectors— where change is occurring, and discussed how these changes might shape the roles of dietitians in the twenty-first century.[8] Her work is summarized here.

Acceptance of Nutrition's Role in Disease Prevention

Future Practice Roles

• Sports and Wellness Nutrition
• Nutrition Consulting
• Public Health Nutrition
• Communications

Summary: Every phase of dietetics will be melded into a new specialty based on prevention, for humanitarian as well as economic reasons. Keeping people healthy lightens the burden on our health delivery system and enhances quality of life.

Influence of Aging Baby Boomers

Future Practice Roles

• Communications
• Government
• Public Health

Summary: Dietitians must display political skills and knowledge of legal issues. They must be viewed as the experts of choice on food issues by the media.

International Concern for Food Safety

Future Practice Roles

• Public Spokesperson
• Communications

Summary: Globalization of food production, distribution, and marketing will be seen, leading to international standards for food safety. This trend will provide dietitians with the opportunity to serve as spokespersons when objective expertise is needed on controversial issues.

Utilizing More of Nature's Food Bounty

Future Practice Roles

• Communications
• Research and Product Development

Summary: There are numerous underutilized food products available in nature. As these foods become part of our food supply, nutrition profiles must be developed and the public must be assured that the foods are safe to eat. Also, new products may be developed and dietitians should be part of the team.

Variations of Vegetarianism

Future Practice Roles

• Research
• Vegetarian Nutrition

Summary: The number of Americans choosing a vegetarian diet is increasing, and these people need nutrition education. Nutrition research will be important to clarify information about the roles of all foods in a balanced diet.

Greater Demand for Nutritional Content Information

Future Practice Roles

- Personal Nutrition Advisor
- Computer Nutrition Consultant

Summary: Both consumers and foodservice operators will need more information about the nutrient content of foods and prepared food products in order to meet specific needs. A combined degree in dietetics and computer science could open the door to many unique job opportunities.

More Meals Delivered to the Home

Future Practice Role

- Foodservice Management

Summary: Computer networks and video conferencing will allow individuals to work at home more than ever before. Food management contractors may set up delivery routes to deliver food to individuals working at home. In the future, the challenge will be to take the food to the consumer whenever and wherever he/she wants to eat it. Dietitians will be an important part of foodservice, not only as nutrition experts but also as marketers and managers.

Year-Round Schools

Future Practice Roles

- Foodservice Management
- School Nutrition Services

Summary: Longer school days, longer school years, after-school services, and the provision of dinner, as well as breakfast and lunch, may be in the future. Such a scenario will increase the need for dietitians in the area of school nutrition services.

Universal Free School Meals

Future Practice Roles

* School Nutrition Services
* Ethnic Nutrition

Summary: The challenge will be to serve meals that are both nutritious and appealing to a diverse group of children. Nutrition education materials must also be developed to teach students from many cultural backgrounds.

More Day Care Centers for the Young and Old

Future Practice Roles

* Foodservice Management
* Pediatric Nutrition
* Gerontological Nutrition

Summary: Working women of the future will need a place where both their children and parents can safely spend the business day. Such settings will produce a greater need for dietitians in foodservice management, pediatrics, and gerontology.

Increased Life Expectancy and "Down-Aging"

Future Practice Role

* Personal Nutrition Advisor

Summary: Life expectancy continues to increase. With longer life comes the concept of "down-aging". For example, when fifty-year-olds look in the mirror, they see themselves as much younger than their parents were at the same age. They actually feel younger than a person of the same age did a generation ago. There is an increased expectancy from life, and with this will come a demand for personal nutrition advisors to set up personal dietary programs or regimes.

A Growing Infirm Population

Future Practice Roles

- Gerontological Nutrition
- Public Health Nutrition
- Health Care Facility Consultant

Summary: As a nation, we are growing older, and the oldest of the old have unique problems and dietary needs. Expanded nursing home facilities will be needed in the future, and dietitians will play an important role in these facilities.

Feeding the Homeless

Future Practice Roles

- Hunger and Malnutrition
- Public Health Nutrition

Summary: Dietitians will increasingly become active in caring for the hungry and homeless. Nutrition issues are involved, as are psychiatric and mental health issues.

Basic Education for Foodservice Employees

Future Practice Role

- Nutrition Education for the Public

Summary: The foodservice industry is the largest entry-level employer in the nation. In the future, this industry will need to provide basic math, reading, and language skills to new employees, as well as nutrition education.

Controversial Technology

Future Practice Roles

* Research
* Communications
* Nutrition Education for the Public

Summary: New food technologies such as *sous-vide*, irradiation, bioengineered foods, and organic farming will be debated in the public forum. Once again, such changes provide opportunities for dietitians to act as leaders in educating the public. Public speaking and writing skills will be needed, as well as technical knowledge to calm consumer fears.

SUMMARY

The future of dietetics is dynamic and exciting. Entrepreneurial dietitians, who see change as opportunity, will be the ones who take dietetics into the twenty-first century. Dietitians must be willing to seize opportunities to market themselves and their abilities in new and exciting ways.

According to Parks,[9] we must develop new consumer-responsive products and services, such as new foods, new approaches to nutrition education, new computer software, and new programs targeted at children, families, minorities, women, the elderly, and dual-career families. New areas of dietetic practice will be developed as new customer needs are discovered.

The profession of dietetics has a bright and exciting future. You will be limited only by your energy level and imagination. Prepare now to be a part of that bright future!

SUGGESTED ACTIVITIES

1. Review copies of the *Journal of the American Dietetic Association* and the *ADA Courier* for the past year. What hot topics are being discussed in these publications? How much do you know about these topics? How do you think these topics may affect your future practice in dietetics?

2. Read current issues of popular newspapers or news magazines, such as *The Wall Street Journal, Time, Newsweek,* or *U.S. News and World Report.* Look specifically for articles which might relate to dietetic practice, including health-related topics, food, nutrition, foodservice, public health, etc. What implications might these topics have for dietetics?

3. Review the "President's Page" in each issue of the *Journal of the American Dietetic Association.* What topics have been discussed? What issues are facing the profession of dietetics or The American Dietetic Association?

NOTES

1. Parks SC. President's page: Creating your future—career opportunities in an era of change. *Journal of the American Dietetic Association,* 1994;94: 451–452.

2. Bunda D. Hospital closing drops for third straight year. *Modern Health Care,* 1992;June 15:2.

3. Bunda D. Number of hospital mergers slip in '92; expected to rise for '93. *Modern Heath Care,* 1993;December 20:27.

4. Schecter M. Getting ready for reform: Healthcare foodservice report, 1993. *Food Management*, 1993;June: 70–79.

5. Maillet JO. From the Chair. *The American Dietetic Association Education Newsletter*, 1994;Fall:1.

6. *Future Search Conference: Challenging the Future of Dietetic Education and Credentialing. Background Papers.* Chicago, IL: The American Dietetic Association and The Commission on Dietetic Registration, June 12–14, 1994.

7. Bezold C. Future practice roles. *Future Search Conference: Challenging the Future of Dietetics Education and Credentialing. Background Papers.* Chicago, IL: The American Dietetic Association and The Commission on Dietetic Registration, June 12–14, 1994.

8. Wallace JY. Gateway to the millennium: How foodservice trends will impact on future practice roles. *Future Search Conference: Challenging the Future of Dietetic Education and Credentialing. Background Papers.* Chicago, IL: The American Dietetic Association and The Commission on Dietetic Registration, June 12–14, 1994.

9. Parks SC. President's page: Challenging the future. *Journal of the American Dietetic Association*, 1994;94:89.

Molly Gee

*Methodist Hospital
Houston, Texas*

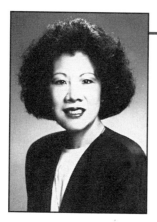

M y name is Molly Gee, and I am a registered and licensed dietitian in Houston, Texas. I was an impressionable junior in high school when I first heard the term *dietitian*.

Food was already in my blood. My father opened his own restaurant when I was in elementary school, so Gee's Restaurant was part of my daily routine, not only as the place where I took my meals, but also a place to work. Over the next 12 years, I was a cook's helper, hostess, waitress, book-keeper, purchasing agent, you name it.

As I heard more about dietetics, I thought that it would be a perfect profession to combine my love of food with my desire to help people. The summer before my senior year in high school, I volunteered in the department of dietetics at M.D. Anderson Hospital in Houston. This experience resulted in my desire to focus on the foodservice management aspect of dietetics and made me realize I really wanted to be a dieti-tian.

I received my undergraduate degree at the University of Houston, then completed an administrative dietetic internship at Oklahoma State University. Boy, did I learn a lot! It was a great experience! I returned to Houston where I was offered a full scholarship to work on my master's degree. Receiving a master's in education was a significant point in my career. After working two years in hospital foodservice, I decided to switch my focus to patient education and taught in the Out-patient Nutrition Clinic at Methodist Hospital. Over the years, I have moved into the management of the hospital's Wellness Program.

In 1982, I was selected as one of the original ADA Ambassadors. This was a major catalyst for my future growth. I soon became very active at the district, state, and national levels within the ADA, and now serve as one of the ADA delegates from Texas. Being involved in professional organizations provides an opportunity to meet so many people. I cherish the many friendships that have developed over the years.

The media provides such an exciting way to deliver a nutrition/health message. In 1988, I was asked to become a regular on KTRK-TV's *Good Morning, Houston*. In 1992, as nutrition became a hot topic, the station asked me to provide a weekly nutrition/health report for the 6 A.M. news. This is a wonderful opportunity to reach more than half a million people each week.

Dietetics can be the cornerstone for so many careers. The diversity of careers is as vast as the number of dietitians I know. Words of wisdom I would select for future practitioners and myself would include:

- Take risks
- Get involved in a variety of organizations
- Be flexible
- Become technologically literate
- Cross-train
- Track the trends
- Network
- Enjoy whatever you do

Dietetics continues to grow and evolve each day. I'm ready for the many new opportunities and challenges that will result.

Index

INDEX

Medical records
    administrators, 168
Medicare/Medicaid legislation,
    20
Miller, Cathy, 118–120
Misinformation, 7–8, 17
Mitchell, Susan, 134

Nanomedicines, 179
National Association of College
    and University Food
    Services, 57, 61
National Association of Food
    Equipment Manufacturers,
    55–56, 60
National Center for Nutrition
    and Dietetics, 71–73
National Dairy Council, 61
National Education and
    Training Program, 23
National Institutes of Health,
    62
National Restaurant
    Association, 54–55, 61
National School Lunch Act, 20
Nightingale, Florence, 13–14
Nowlin, Bettye, 64
Nuclear medicine technologist,
    168
Nurse practitioners, 165–166
Nursing, 165
Nutrition, 9
Nutrition in Clinical Practice,
    54
Nutrition Notes, 53
Nutritional content
    information, 183

Occupational therapists,
    168–169

Parks, Sara, 177
Pascoe, Mary E., 21
Pennsylvania Hospital, 13
Performance Requirements for
    Dietetic Technicians, 110

Performance Requirements for
    Entry-Level Dietitians,
    109–110
Pharmacists, 166
Philadelphia Cooking School,
    14–15
Philadelphia General Hospital,
    13
Physical therapists, 166
Physician assistants, 170
Physicians, 162–165
    cardiology, 163
    endocrinology, 164
    neurology, 163
    oncology, 163
    ophthalmology, 164
    osteopathy, 164–165
    pathology, 163–164
    psychiatry, 164
    surgery, 164
Profession, 9–10
Professionalism, 37–58

Quackery, 7–8, 17

Radiologic technologists, 170
Registration examinations,
    110, 114, 122–126
Research dietitian, 41
Research projects, 41–42
Respiratory therapists, 170
Restaurants USA, 55
Role delineation, 123, 153
Rorer, Sarah Tyson, 14–16, 22

School Food Service Journal,
    56
*School Food Service Research
    Review*, 56
SNE Communicator, 54
Social Security Act, Title V, 19
Social workers, 166
Society for Nutrition
    Education, 54, 60
Soyer, Alexis, 14
Specialty certification, 129

INDEX

Sports nutrition, 5
Supervised practice, 111–114

Teamwork, 161–162
Test assembly and review
    process, 123
Test item analysis, 125
Test item development, 123
Test passing-score
    determination study, 125
Test score reporting, 125
Test specifications, 123
Therapeutics, 179
Total parenteral nutrition
    (TPN), 9
Tribole, Evelyn, 6

USDA, 16, 22, 28, 61
    Bulletin 28, 16

Cooperative Extension
    Service, 22
EFNEP, 22
food assistance programs, 22
food stamp program, 22
Human Nutrition Information
    Service, 61
WIC, 22

Vegetarianism, 182–183
Verification statement, 114

Wallace, Jane Young, 181
Walters, Penny, 156–157
Washington Weekly, 55
World War I, 17–21, 25
World War II, 19, 25–27

Yadrick, Marty, 34–35